THE HOMŒOPATHIC FAMILY GUIDE

Classical Homœopathic Remedies for Common Ailments

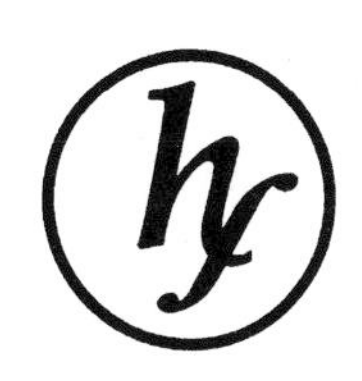

Acknowledgements:

This booklet was complied and written by Dr Berkeley Digby, in association with Pharma Natura.

Berkeley Digby trained in Homœopathy, Osteopathy, and Acupuncture in the U.K., practising and teaching in London for 13 years before moving to South Africa. Apart from lecturing in the U.K. and America, he has also pioneered courses in South Africa in Homœopathy and Acupuncture for medical doctors and pharmacists. At present he runs a busy practice in Cape Town with his wife, who is also a Homœopath. He is writing a book on the integration of Homœopathy and Chinese Medicine.

First Publication July 1996
Second Publication June 1997

Reproduction by ALM Process
Typsetting and Cover design by The Tenth House

Homœoforce Division of Pharma Natura
P.O. Box 494
Bergvlei
2012

ISBN 0-620-20546-6

CONTENTS

FOREWORD

This booklet has been written as a family manual, to encourage people to use homœopathy for themselves and their families for common complaints which are NOT serious or life-threatening, and for which there are not always effective, non-toxic orthodox approaches. Use your discretion when adopting home-treatment approaches, and always consult a homœopath or medical practitioner if unsure.

> Please Note: *This is NOT a comprehensive homœopathic manual; it details the common symptoms of a chosen group of ailments and about 50 commonly indicated remedies. Therefore, if your ailment fails to respond to what appears to be an indicated medicine, consult a professional homœopath. Homœopaths use several hundred medicines.*

HOMŒOPATHY IN A NUTSHELL

The word "homœopathy" explains the basis of this safe, effective and increasingly popular form of medicine. "Homœo" means "like" and "pathy" means disease. In other words, a substance that can produce a set of symptoms if taken in toxic amounts by a healthy person, will cure those same symptoms if they appear in a diseased person.

Let's take some everyday examples. A sensitive person who drinks a few cups of coffee will become nervous, hyped up and sleepless. Thus a homœopathic remedy called ***Coffea*** *is effective in cases of insomnia with increased mental activity. Whilst cutting an onion a person may experience watering of eyes and nose, similar to the first symptoms of a common cold. Thus* ***Allium Cepa*** *(a remedy made from onion) is useful in homœopathy in the treatment of colds with streaming eyes and nose.* ***Apis****, a remedy made from the bee, is useful for red, stinging, burning oedematous swellings, resembling bee stings, on the skin or mucous membranes.*

Homœopathic remedies are made from substances from all kingdoms of nature - mineral, plant and animal. They each have unique mental, emotional and physical 'pictures', which have been discovered over the last two hundred years, through trials and practice by many thousands of doctors.

Samuel Hahnemann was the German doctor who first formulated the laws and principles of homœopathy. He and his assistants took many substances in small and repeated doses, recording mental, emotional and physical symptoms which became the basis of a Homœopathic Materia Medica. When reading about homœopathic medicines, therefore, it is notable that they have mental, emotional and physiological 'pictures' which have become clearly defined through the experience of thousands of doctors over two hundred years .

For example, the remedy ***Nux Vomica*** *has liverishness, nausea, and heartburn which are made worse from spicy foods and alcohol.* ***Nux*** *individuals have been found to be ambitious, hard-working perfectionists who are irritable and impatient and may suffer from insomnia.* ***Pulsatilla*** *types also suffer from indigestion from eating rich foods and also tend to be perfectionists, but are mild mannered and non confrontational and disposed to bouts of tears. If you gave* ***Pulsatilla*** *to a* ***Nux*** *type suffering from heartburn, it wouldn't work.*

When a homœopathic remedy, which has a 'picture' matching a person's emotional state and disease, is administered it 'amplifies' the activity of the inner-healing response on all levels - mental, emotional and physical. This intelligent inner-healing mechanism is extremely powerful if prompted in the right way, balancing emotions, improving the function of the internal organs and stimulating the immune system into producing cellular chemicals which kill off harmful bacteria. Homœopathic medicines are truly 'curative' rather than palliative in a great many acute and chronic diseases. They do not suppress symptoms, nor do they take over the work of the immune system, thus not weakening it as orthodox drugs do. From a homœopathic point of view, each case of disease is unique and can only be cured if it is treated for its individual features. Thus there is not only one medicine for arthritis, as each case of arthritis will be different from any other. One person with arthritis may be worse when it rains and better in hot, dry weather, worse on waking and better from moving about. Another might be worse in hot weather, better in cold and worse from motion. Each case requires a different medicine which 'matches' the 'individual' features of the disease. We will see many examples when we refer to the TREATMENT GUIDE later.

Having discovered the law of "like cures like", Hahnemann then found that, by diluting the substance, its effects were enhanced rather than lessened. Thus he began 'potentizing' substances by repeatedly diluting and shaking them. Homœopathic remedies each have a number after the name, which signifies the level of dilution or 'potency'. Thus a 6C, or sixth centesimal potency, has been diluted (by one part of the substance mixed with ninety-nine parts of water), and shaken, six times. By the time this process has been repeated 12 times, there is not even a molecular trace of the original substance left. The 30C potency is commonly used, and has been through 30 cycles of dilution and shaking. Strangely enough, the more dilute or 'vibrational' a remedy is, the deeper and more powerfully it appears to work. Thus, the very high potencies, for example the '1M' potencies, have been diluted and successed (shaken) 1000 times. For a scientist it may seem quite extraordinary, yet a few doses of the very high potencies can work for weeks.

TO SUMMARIZE - THERE ARE FOUR MAIN PRINCIPLES OF HOMŒOPATHY :

1) "Like cures like".
   A substance having the power to produce a symptom in toxic amounts, will cure a diseased person if his or her symptom picture is similar.

2) When substances are diluted, their therapeutic powers become intensified.

3) Homœopathy treats the person and not the disease. Each person must be treated as a totality, because each will be of a different temperament, and will manifest his or her disease symptoms in a unique and individual way.

4) Healing takes place from within outwards, with an increased sense of well-being often occurring before improvement of the physical symptoms.

SOME GENERAL QUESTIONS ANSWERED

Does homœopathy work?

Sceptics say that Homœopathy only works if one has 'faith' in it, i.e. it is merely a sort of placebo. The fact that it works dramatically on animals and infants dispels this myth. There is no need to have faith in it. Simply try it and see for yourself. Homœopathy is practised worldwide by an ever-increasing number of medical doctors and homœopaths. It cures many diseases which are incurable by chemical drugs. As a result of the increase in publicity about the toxic effects of orthodox drugs, people are requesting safer alternatives from their doctors and pharmacists. A recent survey suggested that 80% of people receiving homœopathy in the UK were satisfied that they were improving with their treatment.

Is homœopathy slow?

Homœopathic remedies work very rapidly in acute inflammations and infections such as tonsillitis or otitis - often a lot faster than antibiotics, provided the remedy is correctly chosen and given in the correct potency. Diseases that have complex origins or have existed over a long period will understandably take time to cure. The homœopathic doctor may need to spend time improving organ function and improving constitutional and inherited weaknesses that are the basis of the disease symptoms. Patience is required. This is particularly so in the treatment of chronic diseases. Suppressive drugs which only palliate, but do not cure, may offer faster relief, but the degeneration will continue unabated.

Is homœopathy safe?

Yes. It is completely safe for everyone, including pregnant mothers, infants, and people with serious conditions. Some of the medicines are potentially harmful in their non-homœopathic state, yet because they are so extremely diluted there are no dangers or unwanted side effects. Indeed potencies above 12C have no molecules of the original substance that can be traced with scientific instruments.

Can I treat myself?

Yes. It is very straightforward to treat minor ailments - in yourself and your family - which are outlined in this booklet. Study the list of ailments in this booklet and select the medicine which most closely matches the symptoms of the person requiring treatment. Wherever self-medication is not producing results, seek the help of a professional. This booklet is intended as a guideline.

When do I need to see a qualified homoeopath?

Although homœopathy is suitable for home treatment of minor ailments and for first aid use, if you have a long-standing or more serious illness, a qualified homœopathic doctor should be consulted.

What diseases does homœopathy treat?

Apart from the complaints listed in this booklet, homœopathy treats almost any disease - both physical and mental. It cures many of the so-called 'incurable diseases', including arthritis, migraines, asthma, eczema, hayfever, glandular fever and chronic fatigue syndrome. It is very effective for most women's problems, and for mental or emotional disturbances - including premenstrual tension, insomnia, depression, anxiety attacks etc.

THE USE OF HOMŒOPATHIC MEDICINES

How do I take the medicine?

Homœopathic tablets should be dissolved under the tongue or chewed, not swallowed whole. For young children the tablet can be crushed to a powder before being given directly into the mouth or dissolved in a little water. The tongue and mouth should be relatively clean. Food, drink, smoking and toothpaste should, if possible, be avoided for 10 minutes before and after taking a medicine, to aid more effective absorption.

What potency do I choose?

For purposes of self-prescribing, the 6C potency (sixth centesimal) is adequate for most conditions. Sometimes a higher potency such as 30C is a better choice, particularly where there are very acute and intense symptoms, e.g. to bring down a fever **Belladonna** or **Aconite** work more quickly if administered in the 30C potency. In cases of recent grief or emotional shock, **Ignatia** 30C is best. In the case of serious injury, bruising or internal contusions, **Arnica** 30C is preferable to 6C. In treating emotional states such as anxiety or irritability it is best to use a 30C.

What dosage and repetition is best?

The instructions on the bottle should give guidelines as to dosage (how many pillules represent one dose) and repetition. In cases where symptoms are acute or intense, a dose of 6C or 30C may be taken half-hourly or hourly until improvement sets in, then every two hours, and finally three times a day once symptoms are not so intense. A 30C potency may be reduced to once or twice a day when symptoms abate. When symptoms disappear, simply stop taking the remedy, and resume if they recur. If they keep recurring then seek professional advice.

What reactions should I expect?

As homœopathic remedies work from within outwards, the first sign of improvement is often a positive change in mood and demeanour, and then an increase of energy, followed by improvement of physical symptoms, in that order. This is particularly notable in children who are ill. They often become more animated and harmonious in mood, with improvement in the complexion and energy some while before physical symptoms improve.

The mother may say: "She is herself again." Very occasionally after taking a homœopathic medicine your symptoms may become slightly worse. This effect will be brief and is a good sign that the body's natural healing energies have started to counteract the illness. After this, the symptoms will subside as you regain your health. If symptoms do not go away, talk to your pharmacist, doctor or qualified homœopath.

What happens if I take the wrong medicine?

Generally if you take the wrong medicine nothing happens and you must look again at the self-treatment guide to see if you can find a better prescription. You can come to no harm by taking homœopathic medicine that is not suitable for the symptoms you are experiencing.

What about taking homœopathic complexes, i.e. combination remedies which are sold in most pharmacies and health shops?

Some homœopathic complexes are effective for symptoms in which self-treatment is appropriate; however, they generally work more slowly than the 'simillimum' (the single remedy that fits the symptom picture). The use of the single well selected remedy compared to a combination remedy is like using a rifle and hitting the centre with a single bullet, or shooting at a target with a shotgun and getting an overall hit but no bull's-eye. Generally if you can find the simillimum, it is all that is required; but if you are unsure it may at times be advantageous to alternate your selected remedy with a combination.

How should homœopathic medicines be stored?

Being very dilute, the medicines are sensitive and should therefore be stored in a dry, cool place below 25 ° C, in their original container and away from strong smells such as perfume, aftershave, coffee and moth repellents. Although they are perfectly safe, all medicines should be kept out of reach of children.

What if I am taking conventional medicine already?

Sometimes both kinds of medicine are necessary for a period and they can at times complement each other. In most cases when starting homœopathic treatment, you should remain on your current conventional medicines until you can consult a qualified homœopathic doctor, who will be able to advise you on when and how to reduce your conventional medicine in a safe way. Homœopathic medicines do not cause any reaction when taken with drugs; however, they may not work as effectively.

What is meant by the expression, 'a Sulphur type' and 'constitutional remedy'?

Homœopaths have discovered that the behaviour and physical characteristics of certain people matches with the 'remedy picture' of certain substances. For example; **Sulphur** types are creative, artistic and impulsive. They are often hurried, irritable and impatient with strong egos. They are usually red-faced, untidy and dislike heat (see 'REMEDY PICTURE' section). The remedy that matches the whole person is known as the 'constitutional remedy'.

THE SELECTION OF THE CORRECT HOMŒOPATHIC MEDICINE

How do I select a medicine?

1) Write down your main symptoms and 'modalities', i.e. anything that makes you or your symptoms feel better or worse, e.g. night, day, time of onset, rest, motion, position, open air, heat, drinking. Matching modalities is very important.
2) Note temperature changes and any food cravings or aversions.
3) Note your mood and temperament and any peculiar symptoms such as irritability, fears or sensitivities, e.g. irritable from noise, sensitivity to draughts or to stuffiness.
4) Study the Self-Treatment Guide to obtain a selection of medicines from which you can make your choice or choices of what 'matches' your symptoms best.
5) Finally, and most important: for more detailed information about the medicines, and to confirm your choice, refer to the REMEDY PICTURES in the final section of this booklet.

N.B. You do not have to experience all the symptoms listed under any medicine for it to be the correct choice. The remedy does not have to fit the person's character type to be effective, particularly in acute conditions, such as colds, coughs, and inflammations or infections. With long-term, chronic disorders, it is always best to find a remedy that matches both the mental and physical symptoms, i.e. 'the remedy type'. Basically the remedy should cover at least three or four of the symptoms for it to work.

It is most important to match 'modalities' correctly; i.e. what worsens or improves the symptoms. For example, you will read in the medicine section under **'Rhus Tox'** that "symptoms worsen during rest" and "symptoms improve from movement". Therefore, if you have a case of back or joint pain which seems to fit the symptoms of **Rhus Tox,** but is worse when moving and better with resting, then **Rhus Tox** will do absolutely no good at all.

Summary: Select the medicine with the most similar SYMPTOMS AND MODALITIES, having read the brief description and 'medicine picture' in the back of the booklet.

What if two remedies appear to be clearly indicated?

You may try one first and, if it doesn't work well, then try the other. In acute conditions you may change remedy if there is no improvement after some hours. In chronic conditions it is best to watch out for changes over several days or weeks. It is best to start with the remedy that most clearly fits the mental state or fits its modalities, i.e. factors which make symptoms worse or better. Alternatively, you may alternate two remedies in acute situations which require rapid relief.

How much time do I need to judge if the remedy is working?

A remedy should show some result within 12 to 24 hours in acute situations, or within days or weeks in slower chronic conditions. For example, if you are taking a remedy half hourly for influenza, you should experience some relief within 4 to 6 hours, whereas skin eruptions, warts or osteoarthritis may take several weeks to respond.

TREATMENT GUIDE FOR COMMON SELF-HELP AILMENTS

ABDOMINAL PAIN OR DISCOMFORT

Argentum Nit: Abdominal discomfort with bloatedness followed by forceful belching. Pains may be worse on the left side. Pains and loose bowels from anxiety. **Carbo Veg:** Flatulence and distension of abdomen with belching and rumbling. Food digests slowly. Weak and tired with a tendency to obesity. **Colocynthis:** Cramping pains with feeling of obstructed wind. Pains after anger. Pains better when curled up. **Lycopodium:** Uncomfortable bloating (see Gas). Pains in the right side of the abdomen better after warm drinks and worse from tight clothing. May have right-sided pains. **Nux Vom:**

Cramping pains after overindulgence in spicy foods and alcohol. Heartburn and nausea. **Pulsatilla:** Pain and discomfort after rich foods or from anxiety. Nausea. Diverticulitis. Pains in the sides of abdomen. Pains are better from walking around. **Sepia:** Dragging-down pains, as if the contents of the abdomen would fall out. Pains extend down thighs, during menses. **Sulphur:** Frequent heartburn. Tendency to pass offensive flatus. Hot, hurried and untidy people.

ACNE

Belladonna: Face is often flushed. Skin is red, dry and hot. Acne: bright red and inflamed. Rosacea. **Calc Sulph:** Pimples with suppurating yellow heads. Cystic lumps under the skin. Jealous person. **Hepar Sulph:** Pimples which are sore to touch and suppurate white pus. Infected spots. Reddish blue discoloration of the skin. Irritable person: bouts of anger alternating with depression. **Nat Mur:** Pimples and acne around jaw and hairline often worse before and during menses. Oily panel in the face with dry patches. Acne with delayed menses. **Silica:** Pimples which remain under the skin and fail to come to a head. Pimples leave scars. May get boils and abscesses. Fine hair and skin. Sweats on head. Nails break. **Sulphur:** Acne, with red irritated spots on face and shoulders. May experience burning and itching of skin. Dry lips. Hot, impatient, argumentative, untidy and critical. '*Sulphur* type'. *Sulphur* may help as an intercurrent for a week or two when the indicated remedy stops working. **Thuja:** Acne of face and nose. Greasy skin and hair. History of warts. Worries about appearance.

N.B. In acne of teenagers or adults, any of the above medicines may be useful; however there are two medicines outside of the chosen group for this book which might be useful: Asterias Rubens: Acne from hormonal problems - red pimples with black centres. Red blotchy skin. Kali Bromatum: Acne of teenagers. Acne of face and nose; may leave scars. Blackheads and whiteheads. Fine rash under skin. Blueish red pustules.

ADENOIDS

(see Nose: Stuffy)

ANAEMIA

Calc Carb: Since childhood, especially girls, disposed to obesity and constipation. Weakness, breathlessness, vertigo and palpitations on walking upstairs or uphill. **Calc Phos:** Tired and restless. Child never satisfied. Swollen glands. Repeated colds. Poor appetite. **China:** Anaemia from loss of fluids, heavy menses. Weak, oversensitive and nervous; everything upsets: light, noise, odours, pain. May suffer from gas. **Ferrum Phos:** Flushes of face alternating with paleness. Irritable, nervous and easily exhausted. **Nat Mur:** Eats well yet remains emaciated and pale; throbbing headache, dyspnoea, especially when walking up stairs; much palpitation and intermittent action of heart. Sensitive and introverted. **Pulsatilla:** Anaemia in pale blondes. Never well since puberty or since onset of menses. Sensitive, yielding people who need emotional support. Child clingy and weepy; wants to be carried. **Sepia:** Sallow, worn out by work and domestic duties. Irritable. Indifferent to children and husband. Aversion to sex. Weariness worse from 3 p.m. to 5 p.m.

ANGER

Belladonna: Outbreaks of storm-like violent rage with red face. Breaks things, strikes out and threatens. **Chamomilla:** Anger and petulant behaviour in teething children. Red cheeks. Throws things with anger. **Hepar Sulph:** Violent anger; wants to strike out and hurt others. Morose and irritable. **Ignatia:** Hysterical outbursts of anger. Easily hurt and offended. Anger from contradiction and from inconsiderate behaviour of others. Anger alternating with tears, sighing and sobbing. **Lachesis:** Anger before menses (see Premenstrual Tension). Over-intense, talkative people. Egocentric and opinionated. Jealous and suspicious. Disposition to criticize and contradict. **Lycopodium:** Irritable and domineering with subordinates and family, yet charming with others. Anger with depression and pessimism. Lack of self-confidence, yet competitive. Irritable in mornings. **Nit Ac:** Anger and resentment, will not forgive. Bears grudges. **Nux Vom:** Very irritable, bad moods, cannot bear noises, odours, light etc. Domineering and intolerant. Perfectionist workaholic. Irritable and angry from inefficiency of others. **Staphysagria:** Cries and shakes with anger. Avoids confrontations then gets angry about trifles. Bottled anger bursts out inappropriately. Feels resentful towards others. Throws things. **Sulphur:** Angry and impatient if kept waiting. Irritated, hurried attitude. Critical and insulting. Extremely quarrelsome and unsociable. Hot and untidy people.

ANXIETY

Aconite: Sudden attacks which come on with great intensity. Feeling of impending death, with hyperventilation - difficult breathing, palpitation, numbness and tingling of extremities. Sudden anxiety in open spaces, in public places, with intense restless feeling. **Argentum Nit:** Anxiety and fear anticipating an engagement; in restaurants, crowded places, open spaces. Anxiety thinking about disease. Anxiety felt in the abdomen, with diarrhoea and spastic colon. **Arsenicum:** Anxiety, with fear about survival, about finances and threatening diseases like cancer. Wake with anxiety after midnight; anxiety worse when alone. Restless and sleepless. Perfectionist. **Calc Carb:** Anxiety about responsibilities, stresses and demands of everyday life; about future survival; about health; on going to sleep; after hearing of cruelties. Feel on the verge of collapse; that they cannot cope with any more pressure (*Sepia*). **Causticum:** Anxiety with fear that something bad will happen. Excessive worrying about others. **Phosphorus:** Anxiety from too many thoughts and worries. Need company and reassurance. Feel scattered and out of control. Impressionable when reading about diseases. Imagine all kinds of problems - worry about trifles. Palpitations with anxiety. **Pulsatilla:** Anxiety in bed, on going to sleep; suicidal anxiety. Attacks of anxiety with weepiness, loneliness and need for company and security. Anxiety in closed places and crowds. Worse when alone. **Sulphur:** Feeling of agitated frenzy, impatience and irritability. Worse from deadlines, being kept waiting, or from traffic and queues. Feelings of heat, restlessness and insomnia.

ARTHRITIS

(includes Osteoarthritis, Rheumatism and Gout) **Apis:** Red, swollen and oedematous joint. Pains worse from heat. **Bryonia:** Slow developing, gradually moves from one joint to another. Pains worse from touch or jarring, after motion, exertion, and heat. Stitching pains ameliorated by rest or pressure. Gout. **Calc Carb:** Joints strain easily and become painful after exertion and from damp, cold weather. Follows *Rhus Tox* well in solid types with tendency to sweat on head. **Causticum:** Stiff, deformed joints. Pain worse on initial motion and cold dry weather; improves with continued motion, warmth and wet weather. Cramps. Sensitive to cruelty and injustice. **Kali Bich:** Wandering pains; appear and disappear. Arthritis alternating with sinusitis or gastrointestinal symptoms (diarrhoea). Joints crack. Worse after alcohol and better from warmth and motion. **Ledum:** Pale swelling of the affected joint. In gout there are swellings from uric acid (*Colchicum*). Pain and stiffness of joints is worse from heat and after wine, better after applying cold water. **Nat Sulph:** Arthritis or gout which is worse in spring and from damp conditions. Reserved and ambitious person. May suffer from bouts of depression. **Nat Phos:** Pains in the joints after eating acid foods, sweet things, or drinking wine. **Phytolacca:** Restlessness, with desire for motion, and worse in cold, damp weather like *Rhus Tox*; but motion aggravates like *Bryonia*. Useful where both *Rhus Tox* and *Bryonia* seem indicated but do not work. **Pulsatilla:** Wandering pains in the joints in sensitive, yielding persons. Pains are worse from heat and toward evening. Red, swollen joints. Better from cool air and gentle motion. **Rhus Tox:** Restless during pain. Pain and stiffness on first moving limbs after rest; on rising from a seat. Pains are worse from cold, damp weather, on initial motion, and better from heat and continued motion. Chronic inflammation of joints long after injuries, blows, strains etc.

BACK PAIN

(see Neck Pain) **Arnica:** Back pain after gardening and stooping for a long time. Bruised, sore feeling. **Belladonna:** Sudden onset of pain with acute spasm and feeling that the back is about to break. **Calc Carb:** Back pains in overweight, constipated people with poor muscular tone. Strain easily. **Calc Fluor:** Similar to *Rhux Tox*. Pain worse sitting; better with continued motion and from warmth. **Lycopodium:** Pains on the right side of the back or shoulders (N.B. *Lachesis* has pains on left side). **Nux Vom:** Back pains with spasm. Must sit up to turn over in bed. Better from warmth. **Rhus Tox:** Most commonly indicated. Back pains worse while sitting or lying and at night in bed. Stiffness and pain when rising from bed or chair, better after continued motion and better from a hot bath. **Ruta:** Similar to *Rhus Tox*, although not as stiff; may be alternated with it on an hourly basis in acute conditions. Pain in bed in morning, worse on initial movement and standing or sitting. **Sepia:** Heavy dragging feeling in the back. Pains during menses. Pains worse from stooping. **Sulphur:** Pains while standing. Dislikes standing - looks for somewhere to sit.

BED-WETTING

(see Incontinence)

BITES

Apis: Rosy red oedematous swelling which burns and itches. Affected area feels hot. Bee stings. **Belladonna:** Redness, swelling and throbbing of part. Hot to touch. **Ledum:** Bites of insects, animals, rats and scorpions; use tincture externally; immediate relief for mosquito bites, bee stings etc. Pale, cool swelling. Burning and itching. **Staphysagria:** Mosquito bites which become inflamed. Give before exposure as a preventive.

BOILS & ABSCESSES

Arnica: Small painful boils in crops, one after another. **Belladonna:** Red swelling with throbbing pain and without formation of pus. **Calc Sulph:** Abcesses that have ruptured but continue to ooze a yellow discharge. Repeated boils. Subjects who sweat easily and may crave sweet things and unripe fruits. **Hepar Sulph:** Early pus formation; extremely sensitive to touch, with sharp, sticking pains. **Lachesis:** Blueish colour with acrid pus which is offensive; burning pains, sensitive to touch. **Silica:** Slow healing power. Boils or abscesses which fail to come to a head. Aids discharge of pus. **Sulphur:** Small boils in crops, in a '*Sulphur* type' constitution.

BRAIN FAG

Calc Carb: Headaches from mental exertion in children and adults. Cannot take stress. **Causticum:** Mistakes in speaking; uses wrong words. Memory failing, particularly in old people. **Cocculus:** Exhaustion after loss of sleep or prolonged hard work. Angry outbursts. Slowed down. **Kali Phos:** Excellent brain and nerve tonic. Weakness from excess worry, nervousness or mental exertion. **Lycopodium:** Brain fag with irritability in intellectual types who loose confidence and suffer from gas. **Silica:** Aversion to work with loss of confidence and feeling of impending breakdown.

BRUISES

Arnica: The first remedy to consider for bruising, contusions or trauma to any part of the body. **Bellis Perennis:** Should be given after bruising to soft tissues, particularly breast. Will prevent tumour formation. **Hypericum:** Bruising to spine, coccyx or nerve-rich parts; fingers and toes. **Ledum:** Helps bruises to fade quickly on the face. Long lasting bruises. Give after *Arnica*. **Lachesis:** Person tends to bruise easily from the slightest knock. Emotionally intense. Dislikes heat. **Phosphorus:** Easy bruising in nervous, sociable and affectionate types. **Symphytum:** Bruises and injuries of the eyeball or bones. Helps pain in fractured bones. Aching in affected part. **Nat Sulph:** Confusion or depression after injuries to the head.

BURNS

(see Sunburn) **Apis:** Watery, large blisters. Red discoloured skin with swelling and burning. **Cantharis:** Given early it will help to relieve blistering and pain (may alternate with *Apis* half-hourly). **Causticum:** Third degree, when chronic. Rawness and soreness of affected area. Lesions slow to heal. **Urtica Urens:** Apply tincture of stinging nettle.

CHICKEN POX

Antimony Tart: Pustules leaving a bluish red mark. Will help to prevent scarring at the last stages of chicken pox when scabs have formed. **Pulsatilla:** At the early stage of the eruption where the appearance is more like pimples, and where there is much itching when warm in bed. **Rhus Tox:** Vesicles itch or burn violently, become moist and crusty if scratched. Itching improves with hot bathing.

CIRCULATION PROBLEMS

(includes Chilblains and Raynaud's disease) **Arsenicum:** Coldness, with whiteness of fingers. May become blueish black. Alternate with *Secale.* **Lachesis:** Cold blue extremities. Dislike of stuffy heat. May suffer from palpitations at night. **Pulsatilla:** Similar to *Lachesis*, having cold, blue extremities. Dislikes stuffiness. Gentle and tearful. Chilblains feel worse from heat; better from cold applications. **Sulphur:** Cold extremities. Poor circulation. Sweats easily. Dislikes heat. Impatient and irritable.

COLDS & NASAL CONGESTION

(see Influenza for Flu) **Aconite:** Best remedy at onset to prevent further development. Sudden onset. Feverish with sneezing and dryness in larynx. Restlessness and thirst. Flushed face. Alternate with *Ferrum Phos* half hourly. **Allium Cepa:** Clear, excoriating discharge from nose and tears from eyes. Sneezing and stuffiness of nose. Discomfort and stuffiness is worse in a warm room and better in the open air. **Arsenicum:** Thin watery discharge from the nose with irritation of nose and upper lip, and sneezing. Chilly and restless; may be anxious. Thirst for frequent sips. **Euphrasia:** Reverse of *Allium Cepa*; the discharge from the eyes is acrid, whereas from the nose it is bland. Sore eyes, conjunctivitis and post-nasal catarrh. May develop into a rasping cough. **Ferrum Phos:** Specific for colds at early stages with sore throat, irritated nose and dry cough. **Gelsemium:** Bland nasal discharge with sneezing. Congested feeling in head with dull frontal headache. Dizziness. **Kali Mur:** Stuffy nose and head, with white discharge. Post-nasal drip. Expectorates thick white mucus. **Nat Mur:** Catarrh of frontal sinuses with neuralgic pains. Frequent sneezing. Loss of smell and taste. Discharge of clear mucus alternating with stoppage of nose. Fever-blisters. **Nux Vom:** Itching of palate, with chills and sneezing. Stuffing up of the nose in a warm room. **Pulsatilla:** Coryza fluid or dry; loss of taste and smell; nostrils and wings of nose sore. Yellow-green discharge. Headache with confusion and stuffiness of frontal sinuses. Feels worse indoors.

COLIC

Chamomilla: Distended abdomen; flatulent-colic after anger, with red cheeks (or one red cheek) and hot perspiration; irritable, wants to be carried constantly and jiggled; nothing pleases the child. **Cuprum:** Cramping pains in abdomen. Screams with pain. Blueness around mouth during colic. Hiccoughs. **Colocynthis:** Agonizing cutting pain in abdomen, child doubles up and shrieks. Incarcerated gas. Gall bladder colic. **Mag Phos:** Colic with tendency to draw legs up. Relieved by pressure and warmth like Colocynthis, but less intense. **Phosphorus:** Flatulent-colic, forcing patient to bend double; improves with gentle pressure or rubbing, warmth; accompanied by belching of gas which gives no relief. Cramping pains. **Lycopodium:** Colic with distension of the abdomen, better after passing flatus. Frowning and irritable.

CONJUNCTIVITIS

Aconite: Conjunctivitis after exposure to dry and cold winds, following surgical operations or resulting from a foreign body in eye. Eye bloodshot. Feels hot and dry. **Apis:** Conjunctivitis with red, swollen eyes. Bright redness of conjunctiva with stinging pains. **Argentum Nit:** Granular conjunctivitis with crusts and yellow discharge. Sore eyes; may have sticking pains. Symptoms worse from warmth, better from cold. **Belladonna:** Eyes very red and bloodshot. Dry; staring; brilliant; photophobia. Pupils dilated. **Euphrasia:** Catarrhal inflammation. Eyes water all the time; thick excoriating discharge. Blinking. **Graphites:** Chronic conjunctivitis or blepharitis; eyelids red and swollen; eczema of lids, fissured; photophobia; unhealthy skin; thick gluey exudate. **Pulsatilla:** Discharge is thick, yellow or yellow green. Ophthalmia, after measles. Agglutination of lids in morning; lids red and inflamed. Sore eyes, worse in warm stuffy room, better in open air. **Sulphur:** Yellow discharge with burning pains and itching in eyes. Redness of lids. Chronic inflammation of eyelids. Irritable and impatient.

CONSTIPATION

Bryonia: Stools large, hard, scanty, dry as if burnt. No urging; stools passed with great difficulty; in young children with irritability and ill-humour. **Calc Carb:** Constipation in solidly built children or people who sweat on head. Stool hard, small in quantity, often with undigested substances; ineffectual efforts. **Graphites:** No urging for days. Haemorrhoids and fissures which burn, smart and itch intolerably. Indecisive people. May have chapped skin and tendency to put on weight. **Lycopodium:** Ineffectual urging to stool; feels as if something left behind. Excessive, painful flatulence with bloating. Painful haemorrhoids. Irritable with bouts of depression and low confidence. **Nat Mur:** Constipation in reserved people who hold in feelings. Stool hard, crumbly, difficult to expel, causes bleeding; smarting, soreness in rectum after stool. **Nux Vom:** Ineffectual desire for stool caused by excessive use of tobacco, wine, coffee or sedentary habits. Constipation from change of diet, during travel. Irritable, efficient and organized personality.

COUGHS & BRONCHITIS

Read this first: It is not advisable to treat coughs, unless they are relatively mild, until you have some skill in the use of homœopathic remedies. If there are signs of weakness or difficulty breathing, immediately seek professional advice (see Croup). **Aconite:** Short, dry cough from exposure to dry cold air, comes on suddenly at midnight. Cough dry, and tickling at night. Great restlessness. Hot skin. The remedy for the first stages of Croup. **Antimony Tart:** Rattling, suffocative cough. Like *Ipecac.* Noisy respiration. Cannot expectorate. Weak and sleepy. Child cross; refuses to be looked at; wants to be carried. **Bryonia:** Dry, painful cough worse from motion or exertion. Head and/or chest painful during cough. Holds chest during cough. Irritable and thirsty. Wants to be left alone. **Calc Carb:** Cough of teething children (*Pulsatilla, Hepar Sulph, Chamomilla*). Loose cough, rattling of mucus, worse from inspiration and eating. Head sweats, especially during sleep. **Carbo Veg:** Evening hoarseness. Burning under sternum. Constant harassing cough. Whooping cough. **Causticum:** Hoarse cough. Hollow cough, with raw, sore feeling in chest. Worse from cold, dry weather, and improved by sips of cold water. Sticky mucus (*Kali Bich*). Loses urine during cough. **Cina:** Harassing violent cough in children with red cheeks and ravenous hunger. **Cuprum:** Coughs till blue in face. Vomits with cough. Cough better after drinking cold water. **Drosera:** Whooping cough. Coughs till he vomits. Worse on lying down and after midnight. **Hepar Sulph:** Rattling cough with or without vomiting. Cries while coughing. Thick, yellow expectoration. Chills during fever. Cough worse from uncovering and at night. Very touchy. **Ipecac:** Rattling, bubbling and wheezing. Suffocative cough in acute bouts; blue face. Vomits with cough. **Phosphorus:** Dry, tickling cough worse from talking. Coughs in cold air, worsens in evening. **Pulsatilla:** Cough worse while lying down, during sleep. Loose in the morning, dry in evening. Yellow or greenish expectoration. Worse in a warm room. Fever in evening. Child tearful and clingy. Wants to be carried. **Sulphur:** Rattling, loud cough. Yellow expectoration. Irritable, red faced, with dry lips. Thirsty.

CRAMPS

Causticum: Cramps when stretching the limbs; at night in bed. Caring and protective of others. Persons who are sensitive to cruelty and injustice. Forgetful. **Cuprum:** Cramps in hands, calves and soles in tense, controlled people. **Mag Phos:** Good general remedy for cramps. Tendency to cramps in tense people who are sensitive to disharmony. Cramps are improve with applied warmth. **Nat Mur:** Cramps in sensitive, reserved individuals who like their own company. Cramps come on after exercise and sweating. Cramps from cold weather and at night in bed. **Nux Vom:** Cramps in irritable, impatient, hard workers who suffer from the effects of stress.

CROUP

Aconite: Dry, hacking, titillating cough comes on suddenly, often around midnight. Flushed face with restlessness and thirst. First remedy for the onset of cough or croup, then *Spongia*, and finally finish off with *Hepar Sulph* once the cough becomes loose. **Belladonna:** Loud, violent, barking cough. Sudden onset with high fever. Red face during cough. **Hepar Sulph:** The 'ripened' phase. Rattling cough with or without vomiting. Cries while coughing. Thick, yellow expectoration. Chills during fever. Cough worse from uncovering and at night. **Spongia:** Loud, hoarse, crowing, barking cough. Dry throat and larynx. Cough improves with eating.

CYSTITIS

Aconite: Sudden onset. Urinary output scanty, hot and burning; urinary retention with anxiety, screaming and restlessness. Child grasps genitals. Thirst. **Apis:** Burning, stinging pains and very scanty urine; last drop burns. Urine may be bloody. Retention of urine. **Belladonna:** Sudden onset. High temperature. Burning and throbbing in urethra. **Cantharis:** Constant, intolerable urging with stinging and burning pains. Pain before, during and after urination; scalding urine is passed drop by drop with constant desire to urinate. **Pulsatilla:** Burning and stitching pain during and after urination. Pain is worse while sitting or lying and relieved by walking about. Tearful mood. Thirstless. **Staphysagria:** Cystitis after sex. Cystitis after suppressed anger or indignation. Sensation as if a drop of urine were continually rolling along urethra. Burning with urging. Urine may be bloody.

DEAFNESS FROM CATARRH

(Glue-ear) **Kali Bich:** Deafness, with repeated attacks of painful sinusitis, and sticky post-nasal catarrh. **Kali Mur:** Catarrhal tendency. Most commonly used remedy (and *Kali Sulph*). Must be taken for a good period. **Mercurius:** Obstructed nose and post nasal catarrh, with obstruction of the eustachian tubes. Breath is offensive. Frequent sneezing. Dislike of extremes of heat and cold. **Pulsatilla:** Repeated bouts of yellowish green discharge from the nose with inflammation of the ears. Useful in a '*Pulsatilla* type' with deafness.

DENTAL TREATMENT

Arnica: To prevent or reduce bruising and pain after extraction. Speeds up the healing process. **Hypericum:** Nerve pains after dental extraction, or deep drilling. May be alternated hourly with *Arnica* after dental extraction. **Staphysagria:** Painful teeth and gums. Rapidly reduces pain after root treatment and surgery to the gums. *Calendula:* tincture may be gargled in lukewarm water as a natural anti-bacterial mouthwash.

DEPRESSION

Calc Carb: Depression with inert feeling - wants to sit immovable or stay in bed. Fears going insane. **Causticum:** Depression with fear and anxiety about others and about the future. **Cimicifuga:** Depression and gloom as if surrounded by a black cloud in nervous, sensitive people. PMS. Sighing (like *Ignatia*). **Lycopodium:** Depression with loss of confidence and pessimism about future projects. Avoids company. **Pulsatilla:** Depression with constant tearfulness and changing moods. **Nat Mur:** Withdraws and dwells on past hurts when depressed. **Sepia:** Depressed, worse before menses with a feeling of indifference to life and family. Wants to escape the drudgery of life. **Staphysagria:** Feeling of hopelessness and powerlessness. Victimized by others. Lack of self assertion.

DIARRHOEA

Argentum Nit: Diarrhoea from anxiety or before an event (see Anxiety). Tension felt in the abdomen. Pains over left side. **Arsenicum:** Diarrhoea from chilling the stomach by ingestion of cold substances. Food poisoning. Putrid smelling stools - acrid with burning in the rectum. Great weakness. Worse after midnight. **Cuprum:** Dark or green watery stools. Violent cramps in abdomen and legs. Summer diarrhoea. **Eupatorium:** Diarrhoea with 'gastric flu'. Headache and 'achey' back or legs. Nausea and vomiting. Thirsty. **Gelsemium:** Painless diarrhoea from emotions, particularly stage fright or fear; stools yellow, copious. **Ipecac:** Constant nausea with diarrhoea worse from motion. Vomits food and drink. No improvement after vomiting. **Nat Sulph:** Wakes with urging. Yellow, watery stools. **Podophyllum:** Profuse, gushing, spraying diarrhoea containing undigested food; worse in early hours. Cramps before and after stool. Gurgling in abdomen with pains. Nausea and vomiting, alternating with diarrhoea. Summer diarrhoea. **Sulphur:** Stool changes frequently in colour, may contain undigested food. Offensive stools and gas often worse in morning driving patient out of bed. Rectum raw. Thirsty for water.

DYSMENORRHOEA

(Painful menstruation). **Cuprum:** Violent cramps and diarrhoea. **Lycopodium:** Painful distended abdomen before and during menses; may feel faint with pains. **Mag Phos:** Neuralgic and crampy pain preceding menses, better from warmth, bending double, pressure, friction. Worse from motion, cold and at night. **Nux Vom:** Cramping pains extend to thighs.

Pains better from lying down. Very irritable with pains. **Pulsatilla:** Dark, clotted and delayed menses; more severe the pain, more chilly the patient gets; nausea and downward pressure; changeable pains; with diarrhoea. Pains better walking about. **Sepia:** Bearing-down pains during menses as if uterus would fall out. Pains down thighs. Backache better from pressure.

ECZEMA & PSORIASIS

Arsenicum: Dry, scurfy eruption with white scales. Itching and burning. Worse from cold and after scratching. Skin thickened or swollen. Urticaria from shellfish. Psoriasis. **Graphites:** Scaley, chapped skin, thickens from scratching. Cracked skin with a moist, sticky exudate. Eruptions and cracking of skin in winter. Cracks of fingers and behind ears. **Lycopodium:** Chronic eczema; bleeds easily from scratching. Dry skin. Eczema of the palms. **Sepia:** Scurfy circular eruptions. Eczema in the flexures of the joints. Itching not better from scratching. **Staphysagria:** Eruptions come on after anger suppressed and internalized. Psoriasis on hands, scalp or anywhere. Pustules break out, then skin dries, scales and cracks. **Sulphur:** Eruptions red and itching. Itching worse from heat of bath or bed. Sore and raw from perspiration. Water irritates the skin.

EXAM NERVES

(see Fear & Panic) see *Argentum Nit, Gelsemium* and *Silica* particularly under 'Fears'.

FATIGUE

(see Tiredness)

FEAR & PANIC

There are many homœopathic medicines for fear and panic attacks. Seek professional help if none of these applies or helps. These remedies are best taken in 30C as needed until calmer. **Aconite:** Fear of death, closed places, flying, crowds. Agoraphobic. Sudden panic attacks. **Argentum Nit:** Fear before an event, interview, exam etc. Fear of closed places, crowds, heights. Panicky feeling with desire to escape. Feeling as if about to lose control. Diarrhoea from anticipation. **Causticum:** Fear of being alone, dark, dogs, going insane, and pain or suffering. Fear for others. **Calc Carb:** Fear of mind and body breaking down, insanity, spiders, rats, insects that sting, pain, dentists. **Gelsemium:** Weak and trembling feeling, with dullness and confusion in the head before exams. Can't think. **Lachesis:** Fear of suffocation, closed places, heart disease, burglars, snakes. **Lycopodium:** Fear before performance, before public speeches, of strangers, confrontations.

Phosphorus: Fear of being alone, of disease, of something happening to loved ones. Vivid imagination. **Pulsatilla:** Fear of ghosts, heights, closed places, being alone, of death of loved ones. **Staphysagria:** Fear of confrontations, of forceful persons. Fear of being attacked or dominated and abused. **Silica:** Fear of injections, public speeches. Fear before exams in a '*Silica* type' (see REMEDY PICTURES).

FEVER

Read this first: If fever persists then wrap the ankles in a cloth, soaked in warm vinegar, also give tepid (body temperature) baths. Seek professional help if it continues. **Aconite:** Sudden onset, spiking; shivering; red dry skin with no perspiration; face turns pale on sitting up; thirsty for large quantities. Anxiety, restlessness, fear of death. **Belladonna:** Sudden spiking very high fever. Red, throbbing; dry mucous membranes. Goes to bed fine then wakes up with spiking fever. Head hot and extremities cool. **Bryonia:** Plateau-like fever; extreme dryness of mucous membrane, intense thirst; immobile. **Ferrum Phos:** Fever with heat of cheeks; colour alternates between red and pale. Dry, inflamed throat. **Pulsatilla:** Fever comes on the late afternoon or evening. Flushed cheeks. Dislike of heat or covers. Thirstless. Moody and anxious. Need to be consoled and caressed. Weepy.

FOOD POISONING

Arsenicum: From ice cream, spoiled meat, juicy fruits or vegetables. Vomiting and putrid smelling diarrhoea. Weakness, anxiety and restlessness. Nausea at thought or smell of food. **Carbo Veg:** Poisoning from fish, vegetables, spoiled or tainted meat. Abdomen distended, full feeling in stomach, belching or passing flatus relieves. Cannot digest anything. Cold and weak. **Nux Vom:** Biliousness, vomiting, pain in stomach, and diarrhoea after eating rich foods or drinking excess alcohol. **Pulsatilla:** Nausea and vomiting or pain in abdomen after eating fatty foods, cream, chocolate or ice-cream. **Rhus Tox:** Illness after eating shellfish. Nettle rash. Nausea and diarrhoea. Swollen glands.

FRACTURES

Arnica: Give immediately for two days then begin treatment to hasten fracture healing. **Calc Carb:** Fractures in fat persons with large and sweaty head. **Calc Phos:** In all cases give 3 times daily together with *Symphytum*. **Ruta:** After reunion of fracture, for stiffness and lameness; alternate with *Rhus Tox* 3 times daily each. **Symphytum:** Use 3 times daily together with *Calc Phos*.

GAS & DISTENSION OF ABDOMEN

(see Abdominal Pain and Distension)

GOUT

Arnica: Patient afraid of touch because sore and tender. Bruised feeling of joint. **Bryonia:** Joints hot and swollen, worse from touch, jarring and motion. Very irritable with pain. **Ledum:** Pain and swelling starts in joints of feet. Pale swelling of joint. Worse from heat. **Nux Vom:** Gout after indulgence in rich foods and alcohol in efficient workaholics. **Pulsatilla:** Pains wander about. Pains worse in evening and in warm room, and when at rest. **Sulphur:** Repeated attacks of gout in hot blooded, impatient people who love wine and whisky. **Urtica Urens *mother tincture*:** 20 drops in a little water two to three times a day for 6 months improves elimination of uric acid from the kidneys and prevents further attacks of gout.

GRIEF

Ignatia: First remedy for grief. Sighing remedy. Silent grief. Moods changeable. Hysterical. **Cimicifuga:** Gloomy, sad feeling as if encompassed by a black cloud. Feeling of going crazy. Nervous. **Cocculus:** Disoriented, confused feeling. Sleepless. Empty and drained from long struggle. **Nat Mur:** Long-standing grief. Sad and introverted. Keeps grief within, avoids consolation. **Pulsatilla:** Crying constantly with lonely, forsaken feeling. Changeable moods. Needs company.

GUM DISEASE

(Gingivitis) **Calc Phos:** Swollen, tender and easily bleeding gums. **Carbo Veg:** Sore bleeding gums and loose teeth. Poor circulation with blueness of legs or feet. **Lachesis:** Swollen, red and easily bleeding gums in hot-blooded people who bruise easily. **Mercurius:** Swollen, pale gums. Breath offensive. Pale, swollen tongue. Saliva flows onto pillow. **Phosphorus:** Gums are soft and spongy and bleed easily. **Silica:** Gumboils develop slowly and heal slowly. Gums recede.

HAEMORRHOIDS

(see Piles)

HAIR LOSS

Arsenicum: Falling out of hair, in analytical, fussy and controlling types. **Lycopodium:** Hair loss, in intellectual, goal oriented, hard-working types who lack confidence. **Nat Mur:** Hair falling out, in sensitive, introverted types who like time alone. Tendency to greasy hair. **Sepia:** Hair falling out, in worn out, sallow and irritable women. Worse after childbirth.

HALITOSIS

Mercurius: Halitosis with unhealthy gums, and pale, swollen tongue. Sweats easily during heat. **Sulphur:** Breath, sweat and flatus tend to be offensive. Untidy, irritable and hurried people. **Kali Bich:** Halitosis from post nasal drip. Tendency to sinusitis.

HAY FEVER

Allium Cepa: Copious watery discharge from nose; eyes watery but not irritated. Sneezing worse in a warm room and better in cool air; worse in evening. **Arsenicum:** Irritating watery discharge from nose and eyes, causes redness. May get asthma with hayfever. **Euphrasia:** Irritated, burning eyes; looks like conjunctivitis. Nasal discharge bland. **Nat Mur:** Frequent sneezing with watery or white albuminous discharge. Sores in nose. **Nux Vom:** Nose stuffed up, cannot breathe. Nose runs; headache; irritability; eyes dry. Itchy tubes. **Sabadilla:** Itching of nose, roof or mouth and ears. Sneezing from pollen (flowers). Burning eyes.

HEARTBURN

(see Indigestion)

HERPES

Hepar Sulph: Herpes very sensitive to touch; may appear anywhere on face. Reddish complexion. **Nat Mur:** Frequent attacks. May come on during fever, from exposure to sun or from stress. Painful; itching, moist, crusty eruption; dry, cracked lips; watery, clear discharge. Pale lips. **Rhus Tox:** Sudden outbreak of many; severe burning and itching sores, often around the mouth. **Sepia:** Herpes around the mouth, in tired, sallow person. Tired 3 p.m. to 5 p.m. Irritable with family.

INCONTINENCE & BED-WETTING

Belladonna: Children who get very upset from reproaches. Children who are very sensitive to being put down or told off in front of others. **Causticum:** Bed-wetting in sympathetic and caring children or adults, who dislike cruelty and injustice. Wet bed in first sleep. Fear of dark and of dogs. Urination on coughing and sneezing in adults. **Nat Mur:** Children and adults who keep feelings to themselves, and don't talk about their problems. Shy. **Pulsatilla:** Involuntary urination in sensitive, insecure children, who cry easily and need support. Child wets bed even if he or she avoids drinking at night. Needy *Pulsatilla* type. **Sepia:** Enuresis during first part of sleep, especially little girls; bed is wet almost as soon as child goes to sleep. **Sulphur:** Bed-wetting in scrofulous, red-faced, hot and untidy children. Sleep very deeply.

INDIGESTION & HEARTBURN

Carbo Veg: Heartburn with belching. Food sits in stomach; digests slowly. Bloatedness. **Lycopodium:** Lots of bloating and gas in lower abdomen, worse from onions, beans and cabbage. **Nux Vom:** Indigestion after spices or wrong combining. As if a lump in stomach. Belching acrid bile. **Pulsatilla:** Indigestion with nausea after fats, ice cream and rich foods. Bloated. **Sulphur:** Frequent heartburn from spices and at times from sweets. Thirst with little appetite. '*Sulphur* type'.

INFLUENZA

Bryonia: Headache worse from movement, stooping or on coughing. Stuffiness of frontal sinuses. Frequent sneezing, often between coughs. Watery or greenish coryza; mouth dry. Larynx or chest painful on coughing. Irritable - wants to be left alone. Thirsty. **Eupatorium:** Aching in every bone; lassitude; sneezing and hoarseness; weight over head and forehead. Bilious feeling with vomiting. Restless with aching. Shaking chills. Desires cold drinks and ice cream. **Gelsemium:** Bland nasal discharge with trembling chills, sneezing and weakness are common. Dull frontal headache. Wants to be covered. Thirstless. Weakness and trembling. Maybe dizzy. Wants to lie still. Thirstless. **Kali Bich**: Catarrhal laryngitis. Sinus headache and sore throat from sticky, stringy post nasal drip. Hoarse cough. **Rhus Tox:** Copious nasal discharge with redness and oedema of throat. Aching in bones and back with restlessness. Sneezing, dry cough, worse from evening till midnight, and from uncovering.

INSOMNIA

Arsenicum: Sleeplessness after midnight; waking at 1 a.m. or 2 a.m. Nervous and restless. Anxiety at night. Fear of death, of poverty or of being left alone. **Calc Carb:** Troubled by worries and imaginings about what may happen; in a '*Calc Carb* type'. **Cocculus:** Sleeplessness after being kept awake repeatedly, looking after others e.g. mothers with babies. **Coffea:** Over-active mind and constant thoughts in bed. Cannot switch off. Sleepless after any excitement. **Ignatia:** Sleeplessness from emotional hurts, grief, shock or suppressed mental suffering. **Lachesis:** Sleepless from excessive mental exertion; particularly at climacteric period with frequent hot flushes. May get palpitations after lying down; worse lying on left side. **Lycopodium:**

Frequent waking, often wakes at 4am. May have hunger on waking. **Nux Vom:** Wakes between 3 a.m. and 4 a.m. with worry about business or projects. Sleepless from drugs, strong coffee, and/or tobacco. Tense and perfectionist person. May get cramps in feet at night in bed. **Pulsatilla:** Cannot get off to sleep from constant thoughts. **Sulphur:** Feels most alive at night and often works best into the early hours. Late nights habit.

N.B. *Lycopodium, Pulsatilla* and *Sulphur* may also cure sleeplessness in these types - see REMEDY PICTURES.

LARYNGITIS

Read this first: If there is any sign of choking or constriction of the passages seek professional advice without delay. **Aconite:** First remedy for sore throat with sudden onset. Take a different remedy if after several doses there is no change. **Aconite:** may be alternated half-hourly with *Ferrum Phos*. **Causticum:** Raw, sore throat; extends down into bronchi. Hoarseness. Worse from cold, dry weather. **Ferrum Phos:** First stages of inflammation (not as sudden as *Aconite*). Flushed, red cheeks. Singer's sore throat. **Hepar Sulph:** Pains like splinters on swallowing. Very painful. Worse during cold, dry weather. **Kali Bich:** Sore throat from catarrhal state and post nasal drip. Chronic sino-laryngitis. Thick, stingy mucus sticks in throat. **Lachesis:** Sore throat on left side. Starts on left and then extends to right. Painful empty swallowing, or swallowing liquids, but fine when swallowing food. **Lycopodium:** Sore throat starts on right side. May have swollen glands. **Mercurius:** Sore throat with bad breath, worse from hot or cold things. Dryness of mouth and throat. Glands swell.

MASTITIS

Belladonna: Rapid onset. Hot, swollen breast with red streaks and fever. Very sensitive to jarring. **Bryonia:** Burning, sore, swollen breast; worse from slight movement or touch; better from pressure. **Hepar Sulph:** Sensitive to slightest touch with stitching pains. Suppurating abscess of mammary duct, with pus; not coming to a head. Will hasten absorption of pus and resolve swelling. **Phytolacca:** Very common remedy. Stitching, stinging pains; may centre around nipple; pains radiate from the spot to axilla and shoulder. Chills and aches. **Silica:** Abscess that becomes hard. Fails to come to a head. Not so sensitive to touch as *Hepar Sulph*. Sticking pains. Fine hair, brittle nails. Sweat on head. Quiet, refined types.

MEASLES

Aconite: At the first stage where there is a dry, croupy cough with sudden fever, photophobia and restlessness. Thirsty for cold drinks. **Belladonna:** High fever with throbbing headache and sore eyes. Face is red and hot. Eruption is red and burning. **Euphrasia:** Eyes particularly red, sore and sensitive to light. Yellow discharge which is acrid and burns. Croupy sounding cough. Maybe alternated with *Pulsatilla*. **Pulsatilla:** Loose, rattling cough; worse lying down and in evening. Thirstless. Sore eyes which stream tears or may have a yellow discharge.

MENOPAUSE

Belladonna: Hot, red face with flushes of heat rising up to head. Sudden and intense flushes. **Lachesis:** A main remedy for hot flushes causing sleeplessness. Flushes worse from stuffy rooms. Wants to take clothes away from throat. Sometimes palpitations and pulsations of body. Irritable and wound up. **Lycopodium:** Hot flushes worse in evenings. Irritable and depressed. Dry skin and vagina. **Pulsatilla:** Emotionally unstable. Moody, weepy and irritable. Anxious and fearful. Hot flushes. Hates heat. **Sepia:** Indifferent to family; spiteful, tired of affection. Low libido. Wants to run away from domestic demands. Sudden hot flashes with sweat and weakness. Tired 3 p.m. to 5 p.m. **Sulphur:** Flushes worse at night. Sleepless and irritable. Thirsty.

MENSTRUATION, PAINFUL

(see Dysmenorrhoea)

MORNING SICKNESS

Ipecac: Constant unremitting nausea, not improved by vomiting. **Nux Vom:** Nausea with retching, worse after eating, better when not eating. Rich foods and alcohol upset. **Pulsatilla:** Morning sickness in a '*Pulsatilla* type'. Worse after fats or rich foods. Aversion to cream, milk. **Sepia:** Nausea worse in the mornings before breakfast and relieved after eating. Tired and irritable.

MOUTH ULCERS

Kali Bich: Round, painful, 'punched out' ulcers. Tendency to sinusitis and post nasal drip. Cracking joints. **Lachesis:** Ulcers on the tongue in people who dislike heat and stuffiness. Wear loose clothing. **Mercurius:** Repeated ulcers. Tongue swollen, pale and wet. Offensive breath. Saliva on pillow at night. Gums unhealthy. Sweat easily. Dislike heat and cold extremes. **Nitric Acid:** Painful ulcers with white coat. Worse from acid fruit. Acrid saliva; cracks in corners of mouth. Irritable person who doesn't trust easily and harbours resentment. Urine may smell strong. Receding gums.

MUMPS

Belladonna: Inflammation of right parotid with bright redness and violent shooting pains; glowing redness of face; sensitive to cold. High fever. Sudden onset of condition. **Lachesis:** Left side affected, enormously swollen; sensitive to least touch; severe pain; can scarcely swallow. **Lycopodium:** Begins on right and goes to left; desires warm drinks. **Mercurius:** First remedy where there is salivation and there may be offensive breath. Foul, coated tongue. **Phytolacca:** Inflammation of parotid glands with stony hardness; pain shoots into ears when swallowing. Neck stiff. May be used as prevention. **Pulsatilla:** Lingering fever or metastasis. Painful ears. Breasts swell in girls, testicles in boys.

NAILS

Calc Carb: Brittle nails which are soft in overweight people, who sweat on head. Supportive, worrying type. **Calc Fluor:** A good general remedy for brittle nails. Is also good for the enamel of teeth and for varicosities. **Graphites:** Brittle, thickened nails in '*Graphites* type'. Tend to obesity and indecisiveness. May be constipated. **Lycopodium:** Nails ridged and brittle. Fungal nails. May have gas and piles. Irritable and at times depressed. **Silica:** Nails peel and split in people with fine hair and fine, translucent skin. Hands sweat. **Thuja:** Thickened and distorted nails. Fungal nails. History of warts. Private type of person.

NAUSEA

(see Vomiting or Morning Sickness)

NECK PAIN & STIFFNESS

Causticum: Torticollis. The neck becomes "stuck" and cannot be turned. Repeated bouts of neck spasm, which may be initiated by exposure to draft. **Cimicifuga:** Spasm of the neck with difficulty turning the head. Left-sided most often. Pain extends to head. **Nux Vom:** Neck spasm from cold, with distortion. Cannot turn head. **Rhus Tox:** Stiffness of the neck worse when reading or sitting and on rising. Better from continued motion. **Lachesis:** Left-sided neck spasm in a Lachesis type. Pain extends to shoulder or to left eye.

NOSEBLEEDS

Ferrum Phos: The first remedy in children who are pale but flush up at times. **Hamamelis:** Profuse bleeding; continues for a long time. Flow passive, non-coagulated. **Phosphorus:** Epistaxis in excitable, affectionate children. Bright red blood. Bruise easily. **Lachesis:** Tendency to nosebleeds in excitable, talkative children. Jealous and domineering.

NOSE STUFFY

(includes Adenoids) **Calc Carb:** Obstruction of nose with sleeplessness. Repeated bouts of colds and tonsillitis. Solidly built, chubby child. Sweats on head. Swelling of glands. Worse from milk and cheese. **Calc Phos:** Tickling of nose with sneezing and obstruction at the root. Restless and petulant children. **Kali Mur:** Difficulty breathing through nose. Deafness from catarrh of the eustachian tubes. **Lycopodium:** Cannot breathe at night. Dry, stopped up nose. Irritable and bossy with family. **Nux Vom:** Obstruction of nose. Sneezes from draught. Cramps in legs. Angry and domineering. **Nat Phos:** Bright orange, yellow discharge. Worse from eating too many sweets. **Phosphorus:** Stuffiness at the root of the nose. Bouts of nosebleeds. Blows out bloody discharge. **Sambucus:** Dry nose. Cannot breathe through it, cannot sleep. Cannot blow anything out.

OTITIS

Read this first: Have ears checked by a professional Homœopath or medical doctor to be sure there is no chance of rupture of the drum. Severe, unremitting pain is usually a sign that there is pressure building up behind the drum.

Aconite: Rapid onset of attack, high fever, sharp pains with bright red ears. Inflammation after exposure to cold, dry winds; burning thirst, very anxious and restless. Bright red or pale cheeks. Symptoms worsen or come on around midnight. **Belladonna:** Sudden onset of violent pain and high fever. Inflamed right ear. Dark red face during fever. Worse at 3pm generally. **Chamomilla:** Otitis during teething. Ears red and hot. Violent pain which makes child irritable; child wants to be held, wants to be put down and held again. One cheek red and the other pale. **Ferrum Phos:** First stage, before exudate; from cold. Throbbing pain as in *Belladonna*. Fever. Membrane is red and bulging. Not as sudden in onset as in *Aconite* and *Belladonna*. **Hepar Sulph:** Often begins in left ear and goes to right, like *Lachesis*; stitching pain. Pain worse from draft; wants ear covered. Chilly, oversensitive, angry. Perspires easily. **Lycopodium:** Right ear most commonly affected. Thick, yellow, offensive discharge. Craves warm things. Irritable and sensitive and averse to being alone. Worse from 4 p.m. to

8 p.m. **Mercurius:** Discharge from ear is thick, yellow-green, bloody, is fetid and foul in odour. **Pulsatilla:** Otitis with every cold. Copious, thick, yellow-green discharge. Patient is thirstless and craves cool air. Want sympathy and company. Clingy. Good remedy to give at 2nd or 3rd stages. **Silica:** Chronic discharge from the ear after repeated infections. Sweats on head. Fine hair, brittle nails.

PANIC ATTACKS

(see Fear & Panic)

PILES

Graphites: Burning, stinging and itching piles. Anus is extremely sore, worse while sitting. Maybe cracks in the rectum from chronic constipation. **Hamamelis:** Bleeding piles. Protruding of piles. Raw feeling in rectum. **Lycopodium:** Bleeding piles; painful to touch; better from warm bath. Pains are worse while sitting. May have a history of gas and constipation. **Nux Vom:** Itching piles that keeps patient awake at night; better from applying cold water. Bleeding. Piles worse after indulgence in rich or spicy foods. Constipation with ineffectual urging. **Sepia:** Bleeding at stool, with feeling of heaviness and fullness in the rectum, which seems to excite urging to stool. May have dragging backache or dragging feeling in uterus. Prolapse of rectum.

PREMENSTRUAL TENSION

Lachesis: Wound up and extremely touchy before menses; better once flow starts. Menses clotted. Sore breasts before menses. Left-sided headaches. Dislike of tight clothing. Jealous. Talkative. **Lycopodium:** Depressed. Bloated abdomen. Heaviness of feet/legs. Craves sweet things and warm drinks. **Nat Mur:** Sad and oversensitive. Takes things too personally. Wants to be alone. Craves salty foods. **Nux Vom:** Irritable and domineering. Cramping pains and faintness. Pressure in rectum. **Pulsatilla:** Weepy and moody. Bloated abdomen. Clotted flow. Sore breasts. Insecure; wants support. **Sepia:** Depressed and very irritable. Sudden anger; wants to hit children. Desire to run away from family demands. Heavy, dragging feeling in uterus. Exhausted.

SCARS & KELOIDS

Causticum: Deep scars, injuries become sore again. May have cramps. Persons who are sensitive to cruelty and injustice. Forgetful. **Calc Fluor:** Scars become painful, hard and inflamed. People who are over-concerned about money. **Graphites:** Old, hard, nodular scars. Cracking and chapping of skin. Tendency to obesity, with sluggish digestion and circulation. Very indecisive. **Silica:** Scars become red and inflamed. Fine skin and hair. Nails split or peel. Sweat on head.

SHINGLES

Aconite: Neuralgic pains after shingles (also Mezereum). Sudden pains worse from cold. **Arsenicum:** Intense burning pains, worse at night. Crusts deep and large, bleed when removed. **Apis:** Red, swollen spots which itch and sting. Swelling of the surrounding skin or the face and eyes. **Ranunculus Bulb:** Specific remedy. Eruption around rib cage. Sharp, stitching pains, vesicles have thin, acrid fluid; burning, itching vesicles in clusters, worse from touch, motion, change of temperature. **Rhus Tox:** Incessant itching, burning, tingling. Worse in winter, hardly any eruption in hot weather.

SHOCK

Aconite: Shock with fear. Cold, trembling, restless and anxious. Feeling as if about to die. **Arnica:** Weakness and confusion. Dull and vacant (*Opium*). Wants to be left alone. Says he is OK. **Gelsemium:** Weak trembling feeling in limbs. Dullness and sleepiness. Wants to lie down. **Ignatia:** Shock with hysteria and feeling of loss of control. Changeable moods. Cries and sighs.

SINUSITIS

Hepar Sulph: Sneezing from draft or touching cold surfaces. Yellow, purulent discharge. Pain in the root of the nose. Post nasal drip, which may cause a sore throat. **Kali Bich:** First remedy. Pressure at the root of the nose. Stitching pains in head. Sinus headaches. Thick, greenish, stringy discharge in throat, difficult to detach. Post nasal drip. Bloody or green crusts. **Lycopodium:** Chronic obstruction; worse at night in bed. Crusts and stringy discharge. Snuffles in children. **Mercurius:** Swelling of nasal bones with congestion at the root. Nostrils may become raw and ulcerated. Frequent sneezing with watery discharge, which becomes yellow/green. **Nat Mur:** Violent, fluid coryza with sneezing, then nose stops up and breathing becomes difficult. Discharge is like egg whites. Loss of smell. May get herpes and headaches from exposure to the sun. **Nux Vom:** Nose stuffed up, especially at night. Stuffiness after exposure to cold. Irritable, angry, easily chilled. **Phosphorus:** Pressure at the root of nose. Polyps. Bloody discharge or nosebleeds. Sensitive to smell of perfume and strong smells. Nervous, excitable and affectionate. Follows *Kali Bich* well. **Pulsatilla:** Congested nose and sinus headaches. Bland, yellow-green discharges; patient chilly, thirstless and desires fresh air. Weepy; wants consolation.

SLEEPLESSNESS

(see Insomnia)

SMOKING HABIT

Ignatia: Smoking in people who have suffered grief and hurt, who smoke to suppress feelings. Very irritable and depressed when giving up. Alternate with *Staphysagria* every 10 minutes when craving arises. **Staphysagria:** Habit in people who internalize anger and avoid confrontation. Smoke more if frustrated. **Tabacum:** Is an antidote to the bad effects of tobacco and helps to eliminate the nicotine. A 30C potency of *Tabacum* twice a day along with the above two medicines is helpful.

SPRAINS

Arnica: Bad effects from sprains, strains, falls, bruises. Concussion and contusions without lacerations. **Bellis Perennis:** Back pain after gardening or long stooping. **Calc Fluor:** Chronic sprains that continue to give pain. **Ledum:** Sprains of ankles and feet with pale swollen joint. May alternate with *Ruta* for swelling. **Rhus Tox:** Bad effects from straining or lifting. Pain and stiffness comes on from sitting or lying, and is improved somewhat from motion. Better from hot bath. **Ruta:** Sprains, with pains worse during rest and from any exertion. Violent strain or rupture of tendons; especially of wrist or ankle. Back sprain (*Rhus Tox*). Restless. Worse at night, better during day.

STINGS

(of bees, spiders or mosquitoes) **Apis:** The most important medicine for bee stings with red, itchy swelling. Stinging and burning pains. **Belladonna:** The bite is dark red, swollen and very hot. Throbbing pains. **Hepar Sulph:** Suppuration of bite, very painful to touch. **Staphysagria:** As a prevention and treatment for mosquito bites which itch and irritate. Sore to touch. **Silica:** As a prevention for mosquito bites in a '*Silica* type'. The bite easily becomes infected. **Lachesis:** Spider bites which cause a blue, unhealthy swelling. Sensitive to touch. **Ledum:** Stings which itch and burn, becoming pustular. May be alternated with *Hypericum* to prevent tetanus after deep wounds or animal bites.

STYES

Graphites: Tendency to styes in people with crusty, scaley eyelids. Blepharitis. May be obese. Indecisive. **Hepar Sulph:** Very painful and sensitive styes in irritable, touchy types. **Pulsatilla:** Tendency to recurring styes in '*Pulsatilla* type'. Red, inflamed stye. **Silica:** Recurrent styes with tendency to form hard nodule that will not discharge. Fine skin and hair. **Staphysagria:** Hardened, encysted styes in people who internalize anger and hurt, and fear confrontations. **Sulphur:** Recurrent styes in '*Sulphur* type'. Red eyelids and reddish complexion. Irritable and hot person.

SUNBURN

(see Burns) **Belladonna:** Intense dark red complexion. Burning and swelling of the skin. Great heat from the skin. Throbbing and pulsating headache. High fever. **Camphor:** Icy coldness of whole body, yet averse to being covered. Faintness and collapse. **Urtica Urens:** Apply externally and take internally to prevent blistering and to cool the skin.

SURGERY

Aconite: In sensitive tissues (eye, urethra) with after-pains. **Arnica:** Before and after, will control shocks and prevent soreness. Prevents blood loss. **Hypericum:** Sharp, shooting pains in nerves after surgery. Alternate with *Staphysagria* after gum surgery. **Phosphorus:** Given day before and several days after to prevent nausea and vertigo from anaesthetic. **Staphysagria:** For surgery particularly to genito-urinary system. Prevents afterpains. Useful after catheterization.

TEETHING

Belladonna: Convulsions; dilated pupils; starts and wakes on falling asleep; sudden pains suddenly gone; delirious, bites, strikes, wants to escape; Acute in '*Calc Carb* type' children. **Calc Carb:** Slowness in teething, or too rapid; gums pale and shiny; fair, flabby, fat; sour perspiration on head soaks the pillow; diarrhoea with green stools; vomiting. **Calc Phos:** Slow dentition with emaciation; teeth decay rapidly; cannot hold head up, must be supported; anaemic; cough with rattling chest; more wiry than *Calc Carb* without such profuse sweating of head and face. **Chamomilla:** Leading remedy; gums tender, red; painful dentition. Child irritable, screams with pain and throws things away; wants to be carried; sweats; one cheek red/hot, other pale/cold. Green diarrhoea. **Mag Phos:** Complaints of teething children improved with heat and hot liquids. **Mercurius:** Excessive salivation during teething; sore gums and diarrhoea. **Pulsatilla:** Yellow nasal discharge and earache with every bout of teething. Loose cough. **Silica:** Teething slow; gums sensitive; grasps at gums. Fine hair and skin. Sweats on head. Large head. **Sulphur:** Rash on face. Redness of lips, eyelids, around the anus; hot palms and soles. Acrid stools that irritate and inflame whenever they touch the skin; will not remain covered when in bed. Thirsty.

TIREDNESS

Arnica: Tiredness after a period of great stress, after over-exertion, or after a shock of some sort. **Calc Carb:** Weariness in people with stocky build, with a tendency to backaches. Sweat on head from exertion. Responsible people who support others. Breathless walking up hill. Nails brittle. **Ferrum Phos:** Tiredness of anaemic people or children with pale faces that flush up at times. Nosebleeds. **Gelsemium:** Tiredness since flu with weak, tremulous feeling. May tremble and feel dizzy. **Lycopodium:** Tiredness with feelings of depression. Irritable. Worst between 4 p.m. and 6 p.m. Tendency to gas, worse from onions and cabbage. Loss of self-confidence. Likes sweet things and warm drinks; tea or coffee. **Nux Vom:** Tired and irritable workaholics. Cannot delegate easily, so take on too much. Insomnia. **Sepia:** Tiredness in people (more often women) with sallow complexion. Cannot take demands from family and children. Worst between 3 p.m. and 5 p.m. Irritable, with angry outbursts. Frigidity. **Silica:** Tiredness in refined, artistic people with fine hair and skin who sweat on head. Long fingers and may be tall. Nails peel and split. Fine hair. May be shy and may avoid confrontations.

TONSILLITIS

Aconite: Face flushed with sudden onset of inflammation and fever. Throat feels dry, raw and very tender. Stinging pains on swallowing. Very thirsty. Chills and fever with anxiety and restlessness. **Belladonna:** Sudden onset of very high fever with red face and cold hands and feet. Tonsils red, hot with swelling of throat. May develop throbbing headache and otitis of right side. Pain swallowing. **Calc Carb:** Chronic tonsillitis in children with tendency to be overweight. Sweat on head. May have slow and awkward co-ordination. Likes sweet and eggs and hates slimy foods. Fearful and cautious. **Calc Phos:** Chronic enlargement of tonsils and adenoids. Child is restless and discontented. When at home, wants to go out. When out, wants home. Likes bacon and sweets. Poor appetite. Scrawny. **Hepar Sulph:** Inflammation and suppuration. Acute sticking pains like a splinter on swallowing. Pains in throat extend to ears (*Phytolacca*). Irritable and touchy. Worse cold, dry weather like *Aconite*. **Lachesis:** Pain starts on left and extends to right. Constricted feeling or lump sensation. Dislike of anything around throat. Pain worse on empty swallowing or drinking; better swallowing solids. **Lycopodium:** Starts on right side to left side. Better from warm drinks. Irritable and demanding. **Mercurius:** Tonsils suppurate and breath is offensive. May be ulcers. Saliva increased. Thirsty. **Phytolacca:** Pain shoots to ears. Dark red tonsils. Pain better from cold drinks, opposite hot drinks. Right side of throat may be worse (*Lycopodium*). Feeling of a lump in throat. Tonsillitis; recurrent or acute. Dark red or blueish-red throat or tonsils with white spots; worse right side; worse from warm drinks, better from cold drinks. Pain extends to the ear on swallowing. **Silica:** Chronic tonsillitis in '*Silica* types' with fine hair and skin and sweaty head, hands and feet. **Sulphur:** Tonsils remain large between attacks, almost touching in the midline. Children who are hot blooded and generally untidy. Thirsty for water and crave sweets. Inventive and lazy.

TRAVEL SICKNESS

Cocculus: Vertigo and nausea worse from any motion, when riding in car, boat, or plane. Seasickness. **Ipecac:** Persistent nausea worse from any motion; not relieved by vomiting.

ULCERS

(see Mouth Ulcers)

URTICARIA

(Hives) **Apis:** Main remedy, swelling which may be red or pale with violent itching. Hives. **Arsenicum:** Specific when due to eating shellfish; welts itch and burn intensely. **Nat Mur:** Urticaria in sensitive, allergic individuals. Urticaria after emotional upset. Worse when heated. **Pulsatilla:** Urticaria that travels about. One time here, next there. Red, itchy and burning - worse from heat. **Rhus Tox:** Burning and itching urticaria or hives. Better from warmth; worse from uncovering or cold.

VARICOSE VEINS

Calc Fluor: Tendency to veins in people who have brittle nails, and tend to worry excessively about finances. **Hamamelis:** Swollen, tender to touch veins. Bruised sensation. Pains worse from standing, walking, worse during pregnancy; better from cold. **Lycopodium:** Veins more prominent on right leg. Tendency to gas. **Lachesis:** Veins more prominent on left leg. Bruise easily. Hot. Talkative. **Pulsatilla:** Inflamed veins; stinging pain. Veins come on from standing or during pregnancy. Blue, puffy feet. **Sepia:** Varices ever since childbirth in sallow, tired individuals.

VOMITING

Arsenicum: Vomiting after eating or drinking. Nausea at the sight of food. Thirst for frequent small sips. Food poisoning from ice cream, spoiled fish or meat, or vegetables. Diarrhoea maybe present. **Bryonia:** Vomiting immediately after drinking or eating. Dryness in mouth with thirst for large quantities. Wishes to lie still and not be disturbed. Irritable, hot. May have headache and fever. Gastric flu. **Eupatorium:** Nausea and vomiting of bile. Desires cold water. Very chilly. Aching in the bones. Gastric flu. **Ipecac:** Constant nausea not better from vomiting. Rumbling in stomach. Generally thirstless. Vomits food and drink. Vomiting of infants after feeding. Inveterate morning sickness. **Nux Vom:** Nausea and vomiting with much retching, worse in morning. Cramping pains. Feels better after vomiting. Sour vomit or taste. Vomiting from over-indulgence in rich foods or alcohol. **Phosphorus:** Vomiting after food or drink become warm in stomach. Post-operative vomiting. Vomiting better after cold drinks. Craves ice cold drinks, and salty. Needs company and likes to be caressed. **Pulsatilla:** Nausea and vomiting after eating fats, rich food, ice cream or cheese. Vomiting during pregnancy. Symptoms worse toward evening. Tearful and clingy children. Thirstless.

WARTS

Antimony Crude Verrucae: Horny callouses and warty excrescences. Corns or thick skin of soles. **Causticum:** Soft at base, horny on surface; on arms, hands, eyelids, face; many very small warts. May have cramps. Persons who are sensitive to cruelty and injustice. Forgetful. **Lycopodium:** Figwarts on male and female genitals. Skin tags. **Nat Mur:** Warts of verrucae on the palms or soles. Reserved and sensitive person. Likes salty foods. **Staphysagria:** Figwarts, dry, pedunculated, cauliflower-like. Large and soft in '*Staphysagria* type'. **Sulphur:** Hard, painful throbbing warts in '*Sulphur* type'. **Thuja:** The first remedy to think of for warts. Hard, dry warts. Tendency to many warts.

WORMS

Cina: Red faced, irritable children with ravenous appetite. **Nat Phos:** Itching of rectum, yellow coated tongue. Symptoms from excess sweets. '*Acid*' constitutions.

WOUNDS

Calendula: Good for superficial grazes or abrasions with raw, bloody surface. Natural antibiotic effect - prevents infection and hastens healing. **Hepar Sulph:** Helps to clear bacteria and pus from grazes which are infected and sore to the touch. Prevents the infection of surgical cuts. **Hypericum:** Good for healing deeper wounds with pains which extend from injury. Prevents anaerobic bacterial infections. **Ledum:** Deep wounds which are pale, puffy and painful, from pointed instruments. **Silica:** Prevents or improves keloid scars when scar looks swollen and puckered. **Staphysagria:** Pains in surgical cuts and pains in urethra after catherization or stretching.

REMEDY PICTURES - THUMBNAIL SKETCHES

The description of each of the medicines is arranged in the following way : First a comment about its main use, followed by a description of the mental and emotional symptoms. Thereafter there is a section of 'AILMENTS AND SYMPTOMS' which first describe the general therapeutic features of the remedy followed by descriptions of bodily symptoms, starting from head and progressing downward to feet. Finally the factors that worsen or improve symptoms are listed. Note that the remedy does not have to fit in its entirety. In acute symptoms the mental picture is not always relevant. In chronic, long-term symptoms, the mental features become a lot more important.

For example: A child has a rattling cough which is worse at night and whenever he or she uncovers or gets cold. His/her mood is not notably different from normal. In such a case you find that ***Hepar Sulph*** *matches the symptoms (rattling cough) and the modalities (worse at night, worse uncovering, worse getting cold); yet there is none of the irritable and touchy behaviour that appear in the description of the remedy. Because you have clear symptoms and modalities of* ***Hepar Sulph*** *it is correct to administer it.*

The treatment of children with homœopathy is effective and rewarding. Here are some brief guidelines. Constitutional remedies have an overall benefit to the state of health, increasing energy, balancing the internal organs and fortifying the immune system. There are four common 'constitutional' remedies that probably 60% of children require. There are a further four that make up another 20% to 30% of children. Read up on them to see if you can identify your child.

The four most commonly used remedies to read up on are:
Calc Carb, Silica, Phosphorus and *Sulphur.*

The next four are:
Pulsatilla, Lachesis, Lycopodium and *Natrum Mur.*

Thereafter important remedies to become familiar with are those that are listed for common conditions like fever, colds, croup, tonsillitis and otitis. They include leading remedies that are frequently indicated in theses conditions like: *Aconite, Belladonna, Bryonia, Ferrum Phos, Gelsemium, Hepar Sulph, Kali Mur* and *Kali Sulph.*

If you read up first the eight constitutional remedies above and become familiar with the acute remedies, you will have a good basis for looking after your children with homœopathy.

ACONITE

(Monk's Cowl/Monkshood)

First remedy for the mental effects of accidents or shocks of any sort. Cannot bear the pain (*Chamomilla*). Restlessness and anxiety are found with most complaints. Tossing about. Anxiety with a feeling of impending death. Intelligent, intense people who suffer from anxiety attacks. Panic attacks with difficulty breathing (hyperventilation), palpitations, numbness of extremities. Feel as if they will pass out or die. Fear of death, closed places, flying, crowds. Agoraphobic.

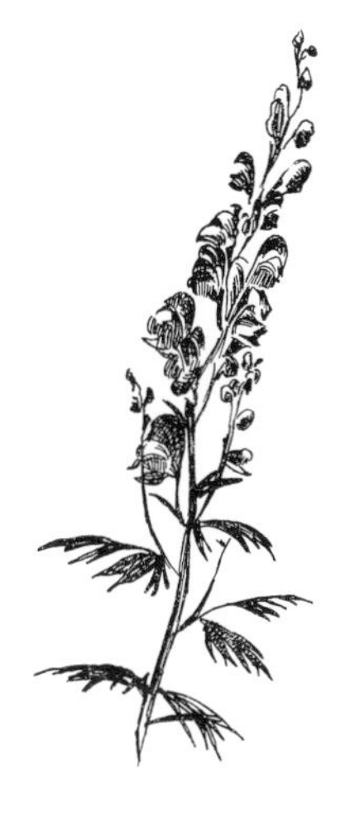

AILMENTS AND SYMPTOMS: Symptoms come on suddenly often after exposure to cold, dry wind or draughts. Fevers, inflammations or neuralgias with sudden violent onset (after exposure to cold). Restless and anxious during fever. Face hot, red and pale alternately. One cheek red the other pale (*Chamomilla*). Croup. The first stage of laryngitis, croup or fever, which frequently starts at midnight with a dry, hot throat and hacking cough. Pneumonia with restlessness and anxiety, and bloody sputum. **Symptoms worsen:** During night; around midnight. From shock. From exposure to cold winds, or cold, dry weather. Lying on affected side. **Symptoms improve:** In open air. Resting. Warm sweat.

ALLIUM CEPA

(Red Onion)

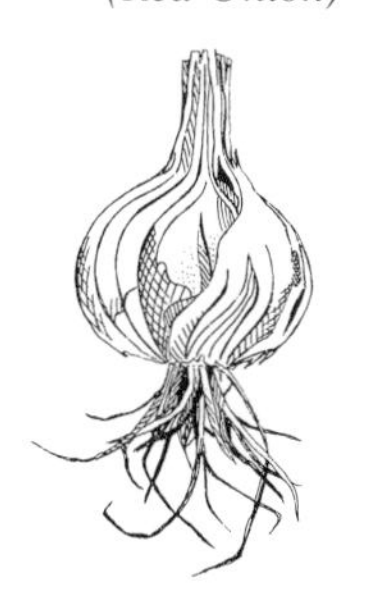

AILMENTS AND SYMPTOMS: Nose and head colds with acrid nasal discharge and laryngeal symptoms, worse in warm room. Catarrhal headache. Eyes red with burning and smarting tears. Sneezing on entering a warm room. Watery and extremely acrid discharge. Hayfever. Headache, cough, and hoarseness. **Symptoms worsen:** In the evening, in warm room. **Symptoms improve:** In open air, and in cold room.

ANTIMONY TART

(Tartar emetic)

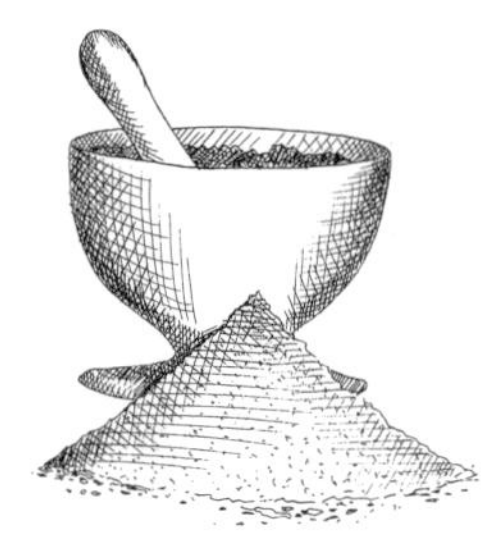

Irritable and peevish, especially during the acute phase of the illness. Child wants to be carried and refuses to be examined. Fear of being alone. Refuses to answer. Drowsy.

AILMENTS AND SYMPTOMS: Children with rattling chests (*Ipecac; Kali Sulph*). Rattling respiration; rattling cough. Cannot bring anything up. Weak power of expectoration. Asthma with rattling of mucus. Sleepiness during cough. May have blueish lips or face during respiratory conditions. Sunken features; cold sweat on forehead. Tongue coated white. Nausea and vomiting with the cough (*Ipecac*; *Drosera*). Coughs and retches. At the later stages become intensely cold with cold sweat yet worse with heat and desire open air and fanning (like *Carbo Veg*); earlier stages are warm-blooded. Weakened state at end-stage disease with respiratory compromise and feeble pulse. Cardiac asthma. Pulse weak and thready. Pneumonia. Whooping cough. Emphysema. Tuberculosis. Bilharzia with bloody urine. Impetigo, chicken pox. To prevent scars. **Symptoms worsen:** While lying. Change of weather. Becoming heated. Damp cold. Milk. **Symptoms improve:** Sitting up. Motion. After expectoration or vomiting.

APIS MELLIFICA

(Honey Bee)

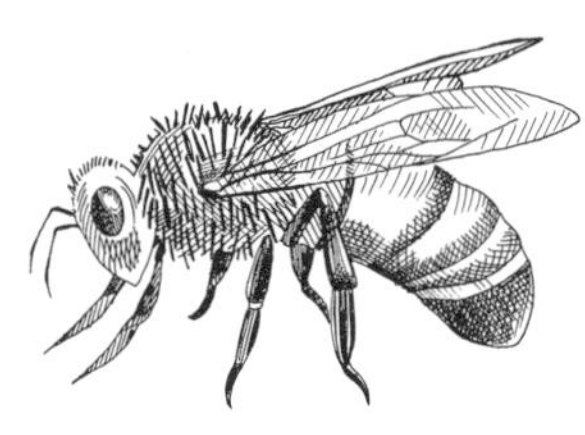

The symptoms of a bee sting are the key to this remedy - burning, stinging, redness, and swelling anywhere in the body. Parts are very sensitive to touch and to heat. Children cry and shriek with irritability or pain. Vital and busy patients; 'busy-bees'. Irritable, hurried and task oriented. Businesslike. Strong family orientation. Jealousy (*Lachesis*).

AILMENTS AND SYMPTOMS: Pharyngitis or tonsillitis with bag-like swelling of uvula and/or tonsils. Throat constricted. Swallowing causes stinging pains. Red or purple throat. Pains worse from heat or hot drinks, better from cold drinks. Pain extends to throat. Thirstless during fever. Tongue, face or skin swells anywhere. Allergic reactions. Anaphylaxis. Hives and urticaria. Shingles with red, swollen spots which itch and sting. Swelling of the face and eyes. Conjunctivitis with stinging pains and red, swollen eyes. Water retention of the limbs (*Nat Mur*). Cystitis with burning, stinging pains and very scanty urine. Retention of urine. Involuntary urination. Ovaritis or cystic swelling of ovary; often right side. Stings and bites of bees or insects with red swelling. **Symptoms worsen:** From heat, hot drinks, hot, stuffy rooms, touch, 3 p.m. **Symptoms improve:** With cool bathing, cold drinks, uncovering, motion.

ARGENTUM NIT

(Silver Nitrate)

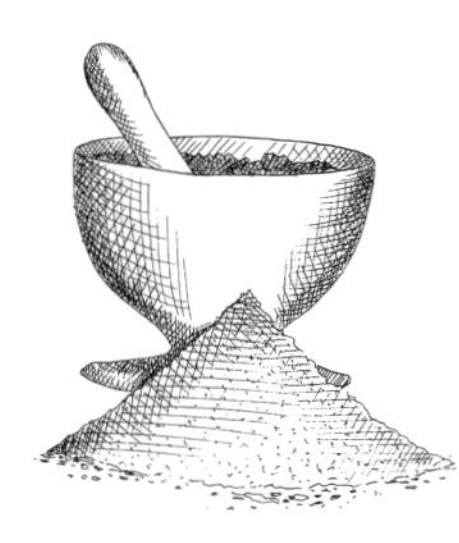

Argentum Nit is probably the most important remedy for phobias and panic attacks. Phobic states from past fright. Fear of driving after an accident, of lifts after being stuck etc. Trembling fear. Open, sociable, excitable, and responsive people (similar to *Phosphorus* and *Lachesis*). Need for company. Nervous and apprehensive before appointments, public appearances, or examinations. Panic attacks. Fear in restaurants, crowds or cinemas (closed places). Claustrophobic and agoraphobic. Face may appear prematurely aged, particularly in child.

AILMENTS AND SYMPTOMS: Problems with nerves, digestion and mucous membranes. Mucous membranes anywhere become inflamed, discharge and may ulcerate. Laryngitis. Stomach ulcers. Cervical erosions and ulcerations. Pains: violent, sticking like splinters. Pains build up and decrease slowly. Conjunctivitis with purulent green or yellow discharge and photophobia. Bloated abdomen with explosive, loud belching. Colitis. Diarrhoea worse when anxious. **Symptoms worsen:** From worries. Anxiety. Fright. Crowds. Closed rooms. Heat. Airlessness. Sweets (which they crave). Lying on right. Cold foods: ice cream. Thinking. **Symptoms improve:** In cool, open air. Cold bath. Hard pressure. Motion. Eructations. Bending double.

ARNICA

(Faulkraut/Leopard's bane)

Arnica is well known remedy for shock or trauma, particularly where there is bruising. Stoical and uncomplaining; say there is nothing wrong. Practical, earthy people. Want to be left alone if ill. Indifference. Fears touch, or the approach of anyone. Weakness after shock, physical or mental. Weakness after stress or

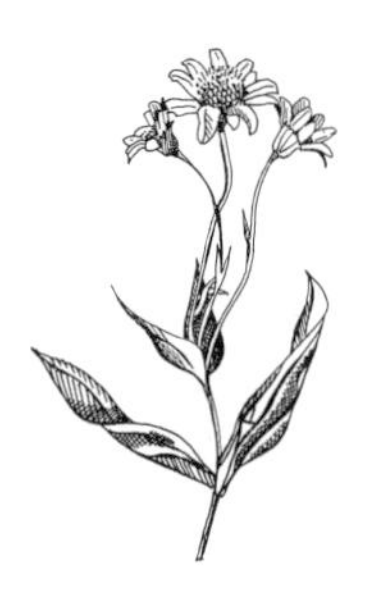

business loss. Sore, bruised feeling of parts. Coma and concussion.

AILMENTS AND SYMPTOMS: Problems after bruises and blows of any sort including concussion. Reabsorbs blood in bruises or extravasations. Useful if given after surgery or birth, or after plastic surgery where there is a lot of bleeding into the soft tissue. May be given 2 or 3 times a day for 2 days before and several days after. Prevents problems that may arise after blows to head. Strokes: first remedy. Useful for any strain and soreness of muscles and back, from exertion. Arthritis with a bruised, sore feeling in the joints. Weakness remaining after flu or infection. Fights infections. Boils. Foul flatus. **Symptoms worsen:** From touch. From exposure to hot sun. From motion. In damp cold conditions. **Symptoms improve:** With lying down.

ARSENICUM

(White Arsenic/Arsenious acid)

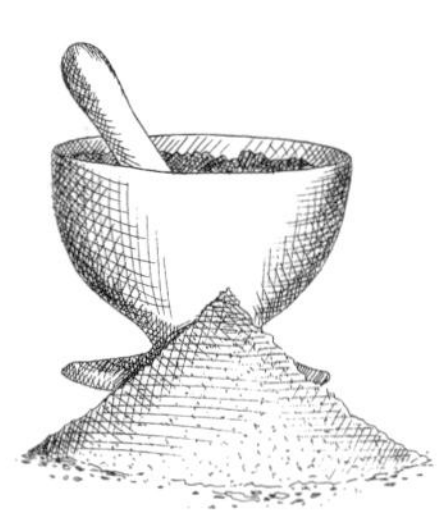

Most well known remedy for asthma and diarrhoea. Anxious, fastidious and critical people. Perfectionist. Dress well. Often domineering and bossy. Analytical, and critical minds; make good researchers and accountants. Fussy children. May experience anxiety about any unpredictable and factors of life. Fears about disease, insecurity, finances, and family. Fears death, cancer, robbers, poverty, and being alone. Panic attacks may be present, with restlessness and desire for company. Agoraphobia.

AILMENTS AND SYMPTOMS: Weakness, restlessness and anxiety with most complaints. Burning pains in any tissues or organs are characteristic. Very sensitive to cold. Complaints often occur after midnight. Adrenal exhaustion. Allergic and nervous conditions. Insomnia with waking around midnight. Inflamed mucous membranes with acrid discharges. Colds with red, sore nose and upper lip. Allergic rhinitis with sneezing. Hayfever. Asthma with attacks which are worse at night. Vomiting and diarrhoea caused by eating bad meat, fruit or vegetables. Putrid stools. Colitis with diarrhoea and bloody stools. Cannot bear the sight or smell of food. **Symptoms worsen:** After midnight up to 2 a.m. to 3 a.m. From cold food or drinks and cold air. **Symptoms improve:** By keeping warm. From warm drinks.

BELLADONNA

(Deadly Nightshade)

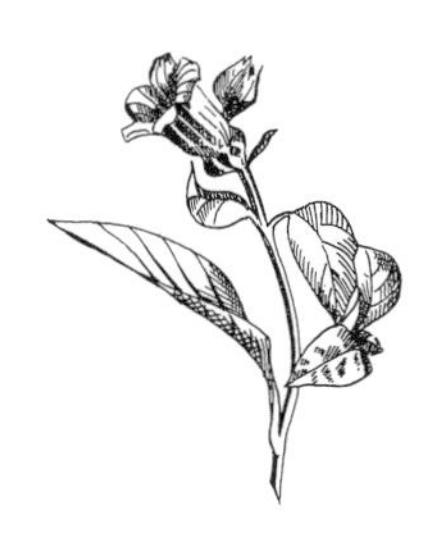

One of the first remedies to consider for very high fevers; for delirium and violent behaviour. Intense and self-aware people, with sensitive egos. Sensitive to being criticized. Children are particularly sensitive to being told off. Reactions after loss of dignity, or after being abused in any way. Anger bursts forth violently, or becomes somatized in the form of violent headaches, stomach aches, or high fever. Manic, violent and loud behaviour. Hyperactivity in children. Fear of dogs, animals, dark, being alone, people, robbers, lightning,

AILMENTS AND SYMPTOMS Sudden onset of fever or acute symptoms. Febrile convulsions. Very high fevers with glowing red or purplish face, and dilated pupils. Cold hands and hot head during fever. Right-sided symptoms. Thirstless during heat (*Apis; Pulsatilla*). Violent symptoms. Throbbing headaches. Violent, throbbing pains. Inflammations or fevers. Intense inflammations with heat, throbbing and swelling anywhere: mucous membranes, tonsils skin, glands or joints. Ailments that come on from change of temperature, draft, getting head wet, or cutting hair. Haemorrhages from any mucous membrane. Nosebleeds. Tonsillitis. Otitis. Conjunctivitis. Swollen glands. Swollen joints. Boils. Mumps. Cystitis. Violent neuralgias anywhere. Acute neck or back spasm. Desire for sour things and sweet. **Symptoms worsen:** At 3 p.m. or 3 a.m. From the heat of the sun; if heated. From draughts. After washing hair. Light. Noise. Jarring. Touch. Company. Pressure. Motion. **Symptoms improve:** With rest and light coverings. Standing. Leaning head against something.

BRYONIA

(White Bryony/Wild Hops)

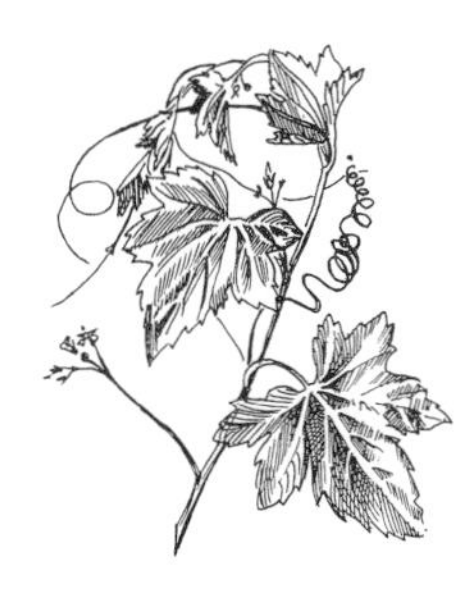

This vine-like creeper secures itself very effectively to surrounding bushes and has a huge root. The picture suggests 'need for security' which is a hallmark of *Bryonia*. The main features of *Bryonia* are irritability with a desire to be left alone during illness. There is aggravation from being disturbed; from movement, light, noise or from being jarred. Practical, earthy people who do not adapt easily to change, and are often over-concerned with material pursuits and moneymaking. Children ask for something and then refuse it. Impossible to please.

AILMENTS AND SYMPTOMS: Symptoms and pains are all worse from movement. Slow onset of conditions - influenza, laryngitis, bronchitis. High fever which builds up slowly (unlike *Belladonna* and *Aconite*). Fever continues unabated for days. Influenza builds up with headache and sore throat. The headache is intense and worse from movement, noise or light. Larynx or chest painful on coughing. Painful inflammations of mucous membranes: head, throat, lungs, pleura or joints, which are worse from movement or jarring and better from rest. Lies still to avoid aggravation. Lies on painful side to keep it still. Pains are stitching and tearing, coming on from slight motion. Dryness of mucous membranes, lips and mouth, with thirst during fever (in most cases). Thirst for large quantities of liquid. Tongue white or yellowish-brown. Hard, dry cough worse from motion and better lying still. Common physical complaints include headache, wry neck, appendicitis, pleurisy (right), sciatica, arthritis, mastitis and constipation. Pain moving limb after trauma. Likes warm drinks, warm milk, coffee, wine. **Symptoms worsen:** From any movement, coughing, sneezing, jarring. During eating. From emotional upset. Heat. **Symptoms improve:** By rest. From being quiet. From cool, open air. Lying on painful part.

CALC CARB

(Calcarea Carbonica - the oyster shell)

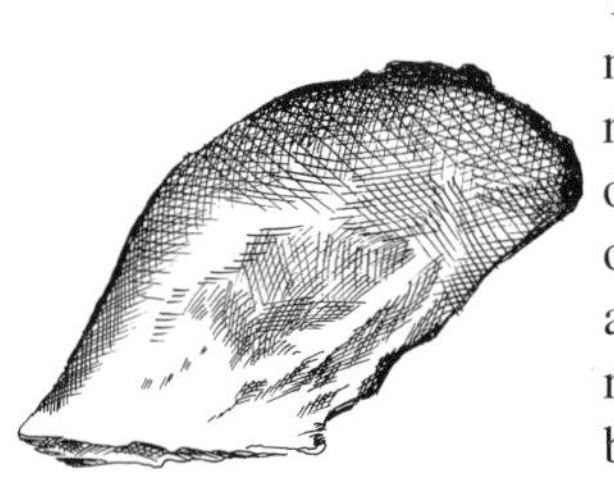

The oyster has a protective shell, which provides a secure, immobile home for the soft and vulnerable creature. This image represents the key characteristics of *Calc Carb* types. They are often homebodies, solid and earthy looking, tending to become overweight. They are protective and supportive towards others, and often very conscious of duty. They dislike change, stick to routine, and are stubborn and unmoving if pushed. They tend to be shy and are cautious in starting anything new. Earthy, responsible, practical and logical people. Slow developers who are dependent on family and home. Responsible children. Often chubby as children. Depression or pains arise after stress or exams. Agoraphobia. Want to stay at home. Feel inert as if frozen by fear. Fearful and worried about everything.

AILMENTS AND SYMPTOMS: Calcium is found in bones. The bony structure often shows signs of strain and collapse. Back and joint pains are common. Pains are generally worse lifting, from cold and damp. Weak teeth. Slow dentition. Bones fail to form properly. Rickets. Affections of the lymphatic system: glands, tonsils, breasts, spleen. Anaemia. Weakness and breathlessness. Tendency to catch colds from changes of weather. Chilly types. Headaches worse from mental work, particularly in children at school. Sweat on head and face during exertion. Body clammy. Breathless from exertion; worse ascending. Desires eggs, sweet, milky and cheesy things, potatoes. Aversion to slimy foods. **Symptoms worsen:** From cold, raw air. Bathing. Damp. Cooling off. Exertion: physical, mental. Ascending. Dentition. Milk. Standing. Looking up. Menopause. **Symptoms improve:** In dry, warm weather. Heat. Rest. Lying: on painful side, on back. Rubbing.

CALC FLUOR

(Calcium Fluoride)

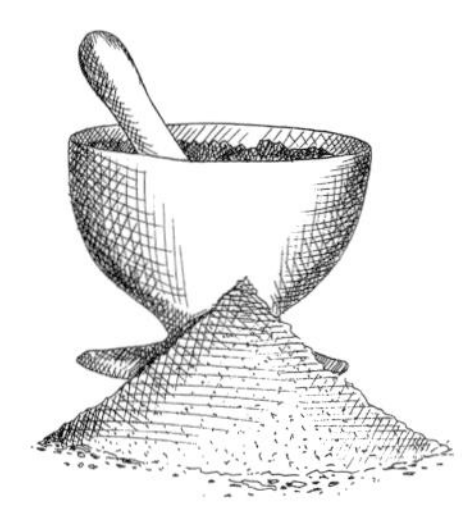

Similar to *Calc Carb*, but more materialistic and less sympathetic. Tend to be hard. Less chilly than *Calc Carb*. Like to impress. Material possessions are important to them. Cautious and distrusting.

AILMENTS AND SYMPTOMS: Structural problems with poor assimilation, weakness, inertia, and constipation, are associated with the calcium component of the compound. The Fluorine component induces hardening of glands and bony protrusions; and the collapse of elastic tissues anywhere in the body. Collapse of intervertebral disks (slipped disk). Back pains improve with motion. Varicose veins, aneurysms. Haemorrhoids, prolapses. Hardening of arteries causes hypertension. Cataracts. Bony outgrowths. Disc degeneration. Arthritis and arthritic nodes on joints. Poor teeth enamel. Fibrocystic breasts, indurated testes, varicoceles of testicles, prostatic induration/cancer and tumours. **Symptoms worsen:** Cold wet weather. On beginning movement. Sprains. **Symptoms improve:** With continued motion, warmth.

CALC s PHOS

(Calcium Phosphate)

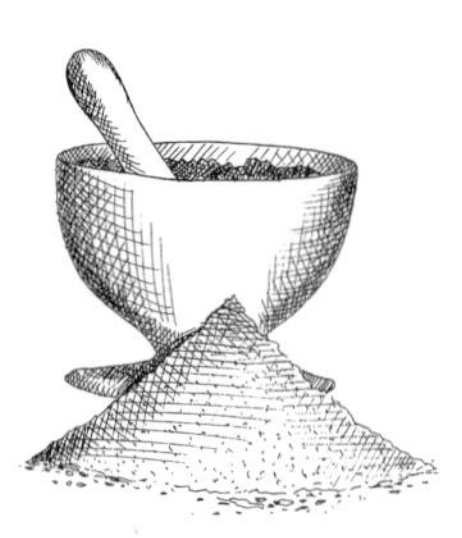

In this remedy, the cautious, protective, supportive and dutiful qualities of *Calc Carb* combine with the sociable urge, and nervous restlessness of *Phosphorus*. Dissatisfied children who become bored and restless. Attention deficit. Not as solidly built as *Calc Carb*, yet they share many of its symptoms. Fear of dark, thunderstorms, being alone, birds, cancer, disease.

AILMENTS AND SYMPTOMS: Structural problems with weakness and inertia associated with calcium, combine with the nervous depletion of Phosphorus. Malassimilation. Poor physical development. Bones fail to develop (*Calc Carb.*) Slow learning to walk. Slow teething. Teeth decay. Spinal curvature. Coldness or soreness in spots. Nose cold. Crawling and numbness of skin (M.E. or Myalgic Encephalo-myelitis). Anaemia. Chronic tonsillitis. Swollen glands. Mucous in larynx. Frequent colds. Desire for salty, spicy foods, and smoked or cured meat: bacon and pork. **Symptoms worsen:** From weather changes. Draughts. Cold; melting snow. Dentition. Mental exertion. Lifting. **Symptoms improve:** In summer. Warm dry weather. Lying down.

CALC SULPH

(Calcium Sulphate/Plaster of Paris)

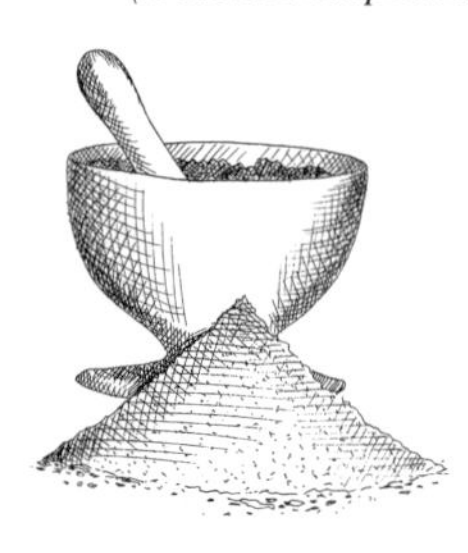

'Plaster of Paris' is a compound, which when moistened and dried, become hard and rigid. The '*Calc Sulph* type' may be hard emotionally, as a protective mechanism against lack of self confidence. Egocentric need for appreciation (*Sulphur*) therefore very susceptible to sibling jealousy as child. Complains of not being appreciated. Dogmatic opinions with anger toward those who do not agree with him. Quarrelsome. Cautious. Protective of others. Manic depression.

AILMENTS AND SYMPTOMS: Hotter and more plethoric (red faced) than the other calcium compounds. Squarish earthy body. Sweat easily on face and body. Pustules or acne of face. Heartburn, digestive complaints, diarrhoea, burnings, suppurations, discharges, boils, abscesses, fistulae and skin problems (*Sulphur*). Poor skin. Eczema. Discharges from the mucous membranes are yellow. Sinus and catarrh with headaches. Chronic hoarseness.

Croupy cough. Likes sweets, unripe fruit, green apples. **Symptoms worsen:** In draughts. **Symptoms improve:** In open air.

CANTHARIS
(Spanish Fly)

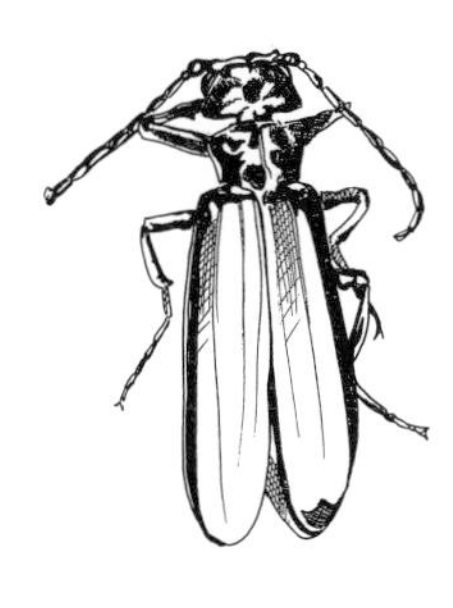

The mental symptoms of *Cantharis* are a direct reflection of the physical, inflamed, violent and destructive. Anger or great irritability. Negative manifestations of pride, with impulses to criticize and contradict occur. Contemptuous. Anger and resentment may be internalized producing inflammations of the internal organs and tissues. *Cantharis* has cured cases of mania which resemble *Stramonium*. Delirium with violence, rage and often with sexual mania is described in our literature. Fear of mirrors and water during mania. Sometimes very sexual. Sexual dreams. Anxiety about health.

AILMENTS AND SYMPTOMS: *Cantharis* is well known for its ability to relieve the acute pains and inflammation of cystitis. *Cantharis* or Spanish Fly, was known as an aphrodisiac. When taken in small doses it causes a sort of voluptuous irritation of the urethra and genitals. In larger doses it violently irritates the tissues and mucous membranes with which it comes into contact, outside and within the body, causing vesicular lesions, burning and itching. It brings about destructive inflammatory reactions in kidney, bladder and bowels. Thus it is useful in the treatment of colitis, nephritis, cystitis; burns with blistering and burning pains; and painful herpes genitalis. Relieves the severe pain following a burn, and promotes healing (*Urtica Urens*). Skin inflamed. Vesicles with itching and great burning. Erysipelas. Symptoms may come on very rapidly (*Belladonna*; *Aconite*) progressing rapidly into severe, destructive pathology. Burning pains with any conditions. Burning pains may be found in the brain, eyes, larynx, skin, lungs, gastro-intestinal tract or genito-urinary system. Cystitis, interstitial cystitis, urethritis, pyelonephritis with tenesmus. Great burning before, after, but especially during urination; each drop passes as if scalding water. Clots of blood in urine. Burning and itching of labia, worse from urination. The irritation of the genitals may cause heightened sexual feelings. **Symptoms worsen:** Before, during and after urination. From cold. Coffee. **Symptoms improve:** By warmth. Cold applications improve painful skin lesions and burns.

CAUSTICUM

(Distillate of Potassium Sulphate and Cacium Carbonate)

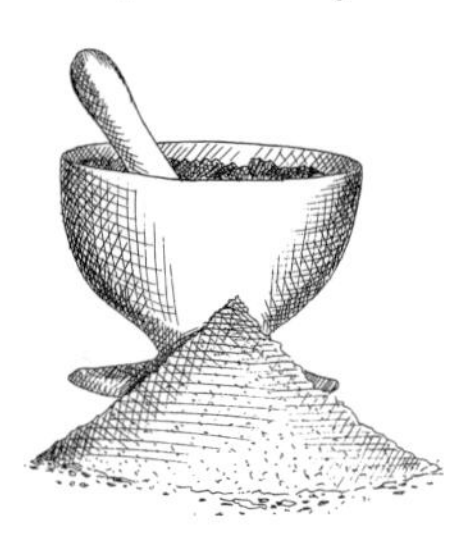

This remedy is made from "marble" which has been put through a special process. Think of marble statues and 'heroes' when you learn about the *Causticum* character. Compassionate and sympathetic people. Concerned about human welfare and ecology. Upset and angry about inhumanity, and the suffering of children and animals. Follow humane causes. Courageous and heroic in the face of adversity. They tend to worry too much about others, about family and children. Fear pain and hate seeing violence. Squeamish. Fear of being alone, of dark, and of dogs. Fear that something terrible will happen. Mental dullness and forgetfulness. Memory loss, particularly in old people. Anxiety and depression, with a feeling of impending breakdown, of insanity. Panic attacks.

AILMENTS AND SYMPTOMS: Loss of control of mind and body. Collapse. Nervous diseases with weakness and paralysis of muscles. Involuntary urination, ptosis of eyelids, awkwardness of limbs. Bed-wetting. Tremors of the limbs. Cramps and spasms. Contraction of tendons. Depuytren's or 'trigger finger'. Neck and back spasm. Multiple sclerosis. Bell's palsy. Rheumatic complaints in cold, dry weather. Soreness and rawness of larynx and trachea. Hoarseness. Croup. Catarrhal inflammation of larynx (*Kali Bich*; *Ferrum Phos; Euphrasia*). Poor digestion. Inability to digest wheat. Coeliac disease. Prolapse of organs. Likes smoked meats. Dislikes sour things. Worse from bread and sour fruits. **Symptoms worsen:** From dry, cold winds. In clear, fine weather, cold air. From motion of carriage. **Symptoms improve:** Warmth. Wet weather. Drinking

CARBO VEG

(Vegetable Charcoal)

Pessimistic people who lack confidence. Look on the dark side. Lazy and sluggish.

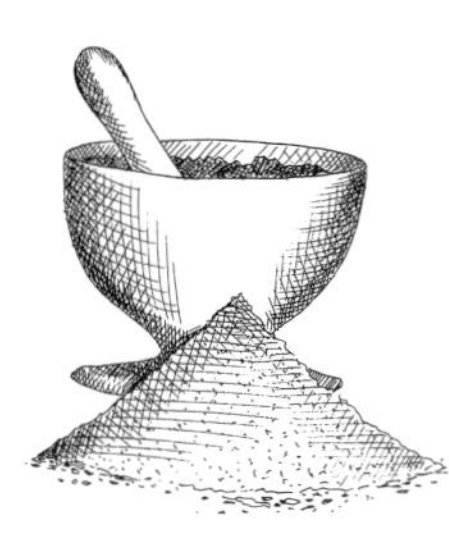

AILMENTS AND SYMPTOMS: Useful medicine for bloatedness, belching, and heartburn. Uncomfortable gas better after passing flatus. Counteracts mild food poisoning when caused by fish. Revives where there is weakness and collapse. Faint and breathless. Hoarseness, rough throat without pain. Loss of voice in evenings. Circulatory problems. Blue, cold extremities. Varicose veins and ulcers with black or blue patches of skin. Ailments following cold damp weather. Chilly but likes window open. **Symptoms worsen:** After eating fatty foods. During damp weather. At night. In cold, frosty weather. **Symptoms improve:** In cool air and after belching.

CHAMOMILLA

(Chamomile)

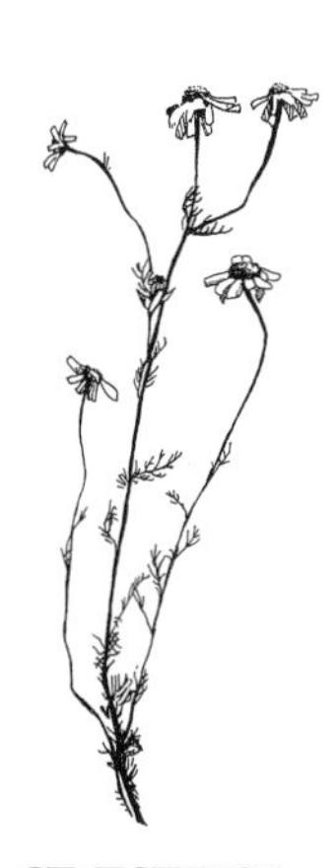

Irritable, whiny, complaining kids. Infants who always cry, even during sleep, especially while teething, or toothache. Desire to be carried. Capriciousness: they want something, demand it, when they get it they throw it away. Children with colic who scream until picked up and carried. One cheek red the other pale.

AILMENTS AND SYMPTOMS: Ailments that arise from teething: otitis, coryza, cough and diarrhoea. Diarrhoea like chopped, green spinach. Arthritic inflammation of joints. Hot and bothered look. Pains are unbearable. Give for pains of teething half hourly till relieved. **Symptoms improve:** Being carried. In mild weather. **Symptoms worsen:** During dentition. Night. From anger. Heat. Coffee.

CIMICIFUGA

(Black Snake Root/Actaea Racemosa)

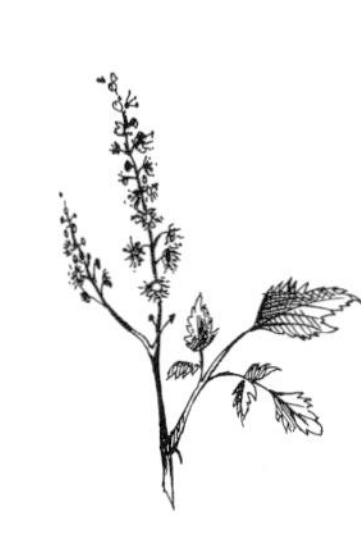

The *Cimicifuga* patient is excitable, extrovert, and forceful. Usually we find great talkativeness with jumping from subject to subject. The emotions are vivid and hysterical in nature. The patient seems vivacious yet may complain of feelings of depression - as if surrounded by a black cloud. Constant sighing (*Ignatia*). Gloomy feeling. Premenstrual tension. Sometimes have strong fears and phobias: of death, insanity, injury, rats or mice.

AILMENTS AND SYMPTOMS: The physical symptoms of *Cimicifuga* often involve spasms of muscles: neck or back spasm.

Rheumatic complaints with shooting pains downwards or stitching pains that go all over. Complaints related to menstrual disorders, climacteric, postnatal period. Painful menses with pains extending into the thighs. The more profuse the flow, the greater the suffering. Premenstrual syndrome. Cramping pain in uterus, compelling to bend. Labour-like pain in small of back. Prolapse of uterus. Habitual abortion (third month). Rheumatic affections during menopause. Ailments during pregnancy: nausea, vomiting, sleeplessness, shooting pains, sadness. **Symptoms worsen:** Before and during menses. Emotions. Alcohol. Night. Change of weather. Heat, cold damp, draught. Sitting. Motion. **Symptoms improve:** With warm wraps. Open air. Pressure. Eating. Continued motion (*Rhus Tox.)*

CINA
(Worm Seed)

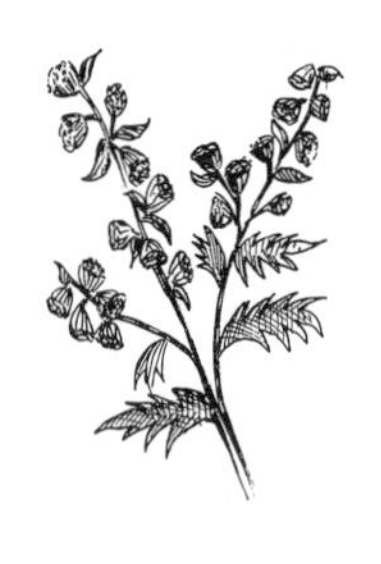

Children who are big, and fat having rosy cheeks, or emaciated, with ravenous hunger. They stiffen out and may convulse when looked at, during cough or when they become cross. Very nervy and irritable child. Sour smell of body, especially in children. Desire to be carried. Angry striking.

AILMENTS AND SYMPTOMS: Coughs with retching, worse during sleep. Limbs jerk during cough. Worms. Grinding teeth. Picking nose constantly. **Symptoms worsen:** From touch. Vexation. Looked at. During sleep. Staring. Yawning. Full moon. In sun. **Symptoms improve:** When lying on abdomen. Wiping eyes. Motion. Shaking head. Rocking.

COCCULUS
(Indian Cockle)

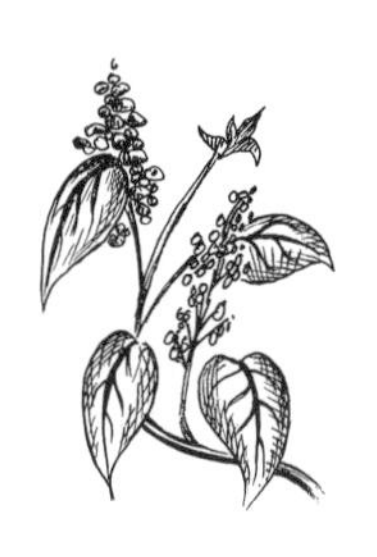

Often self-sacrificing people (Florence Nightingales) who serve others in need. Motivated by feelings of duty to family, children or others (*Sepia*). Worries about others. Exhausted by giving. May eventually become angry and overwrought at demands of others. Easily offended; angry from contradiction or rudeness. Suppressed anger and resentment. Share similarities with *Sepia, Nux Vom* and *Staphysagria*. Become slowed down, dull and confused. React slowly. Nerves on edge, worse from sensual impressions: noise or conversation. Unmarried women; childless women; romantic, sensitive girls; bookworms.

AILMENTS AND SYMPTOMS: The most well known remedy for travel sickness, with nausea and vomiting. Vertigo and nausea from travel by boat or in a car. Feel worse from watching passing scenery. Confusion and weakness from eating or drinking. Nausea at sight or smell of food. Hang-overs. Chronic fatigue syndrome. Multiple sclerosis. Breakdown of the nervous system, with numbness and paralysis of parts, e.g. tongue. Paralytic weakness with numbness and trembling. Awkward limbs. Cramps and contractures of the muscles. Numbness of hands and feet. Insomnia from being awake for long periods, looking after others, from business worries. Nursing mothers. Wake from the slightest noise (*Nux Vom; Phosphorus*). Desire for beer. Old inebriates. **Symptoms worsen:** While travelling in a car or boat. Loss of sleep. Touch or jarring. Noise. Exertion. Coffee. Emotions. **Symptoms improve:** With resting. Lying. Sitting.

COFFEA
(Coffee)

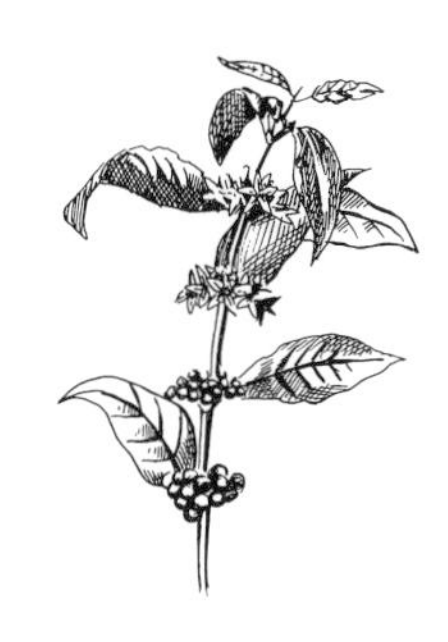

This remedy is known for its use in the treatment of insomnia. Initially coffee causes wakefulness and improved alertness; however if taken to excess it results in nervousness, restlessness, and over-sensitivity to stimuli. The '*Coffea* type' is highly sensitive, nervous and over-reactive. Excitement of the mind. The perceptions are acute, the mind is excitable: rapid thinking. The mind races uncontrollably, particularly on lying down to sleep.

AILMENTS AND SYMPTOMS: Bad effects from any surprise, stimulation or excitement. Great sensitivity to noise, taste, and other stimuli. Sleeplessness from grief. Overexcited children. **Symptoms worsen:** From mental exertion. Night. Noise. Excitement. **Symptoms improve:** After rest. From warmth.

COLOCYNTHIS
(Squirting/Bitter Cucumber)

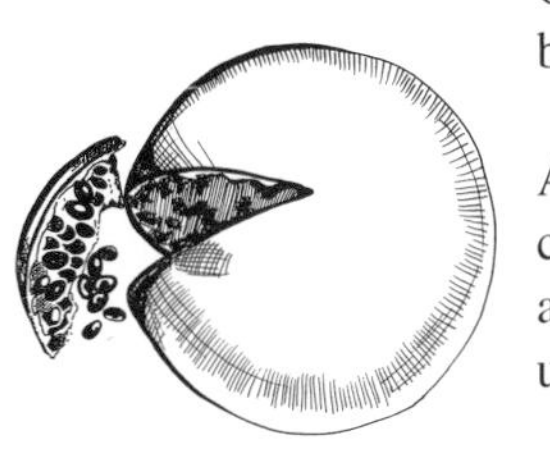

One of the main remedies for colic with cramping pains improved by drawing up the legs and putting pressure on the abdomen.

AILMENTS AND SYMPTOMS: Colic of newborns. Anger with colic, or colic and cramping pains that come on after feeling angry or indignant. Gallbladder colic (gallstones). Colic of the ureter (kidney stones), or of the uterus (dysmenorrhoea).

Colocynthis is also useful in cases of neuralgia and sciatica, often right sided. Abdominal pain. Cholecystitis. Painful menses. Facial neuralgia. Gastroenteritis. Headache. Irritable bowel syndrome. Kidney stones. Neuralgia. Sciatica. **Symptoms worsen:** From anger or upset. At night. While lying extended. After eating or drinking. **Symptoms improve:** With pressure on the abdomen. Lying on abdomen. Bending double. Gentle motion.

CUPRUM MET

(Copper)

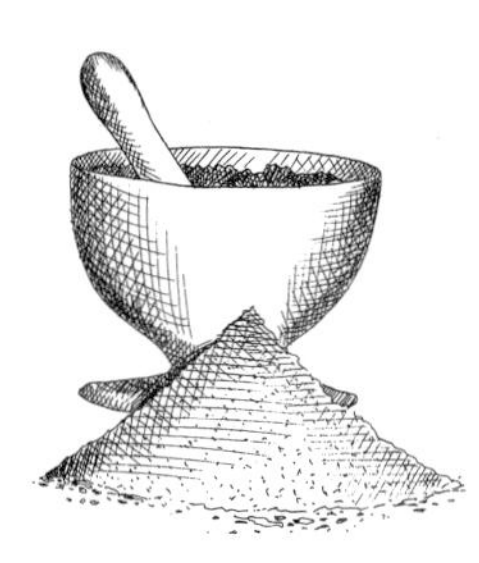

The *Cuprum* patient has been described as having intense emotions or impulses which are strongly suppressed. To maintain control over strong inner emotions, the patient rigidly closes down every expression. This makes the patient appear absolutely closed. Spasms, cramps and convulsions occur from release of this rigid tension. Eventually, the patient closes so much that he becomes dull and slow, even to the point of senility.

AILMENTS AND SYMPTOMS: Cramps and spasms of the respiratory system (asthma), the gastrointestinal system (hiccoughs, colic and spasmodic vomiting), the musculoskeletal system (leg cramps), but most importantly in the nervous system in the form of convulsions. *Cuprum* is the foremost specific remedy for seizure disorders and epilepsy. Convulsion worse at night, worse during pregnancy or menses, from vexation or excited emotions, during sleep, or from getting wet. Epilepsy with aura in solar plexus. Colic, spasms and cramps in abdomen. Facial tics or grimaces. Vomits before convulsions. Convulsions begin in the hands and spread to body. Twitches of the muscles, worse in fingers and toes. Cyanosis: blue in face. Coughing in severe, suffocative paroxysms. Goes blue in the face. Paroxysms of cough, very severe. Whooping cough. Cough and asthma may become worse around 3 a.m. Relieved by cold drinks. Cramps of the muscles, especially legs, feet and hands. **Symptoms worsen:** From emotions; anger, fright. Suppressions, particularly suppressed eruptions like measles. From overwork. Motion. Touch. Loss of sleep. Hot weather. Vomiting. Raising arms. Before menses. **Symptoms improve:** With consumption of cold drinks. Pressure over heart.

DROSERA

(Sundew - carnivorous plant from marshy districts)

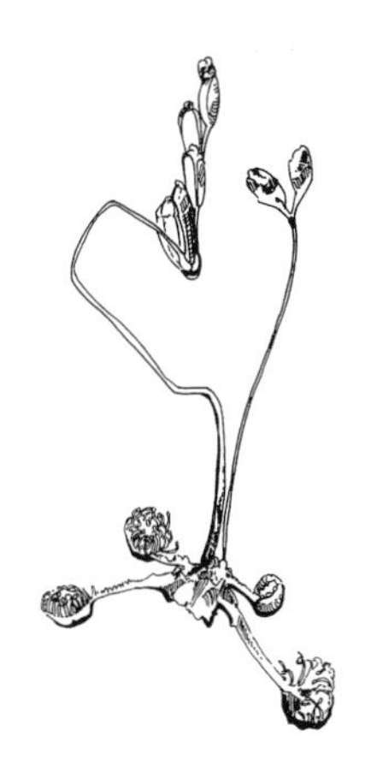

Persecuted feelings. Easily angered; a trifle makes him beside himself. Imagines he was being teased or deceived purposely by others. Restless and anxious.

AILMENTS AND SYMPTOMS: Whooping cough or chronic irritating cough. Dryness and irritation of throat or larynx, provoking cough. Violent paroxysms of coughing so that the person cannot catch his or her breath, and may become blue in the face (*Cuprum*). Vomiting from the cough. Cough worse after midnight and lying down. Painful cough; the patient must hold his chest when coughing. **Symptoms worsen:** After midnight. On lying down. Warmth. Talking. Laughing. After measles. **Symptoms improve:** With pressure. Open air. Walking. Sitting up.

EUPATORIUM

(Boneset)

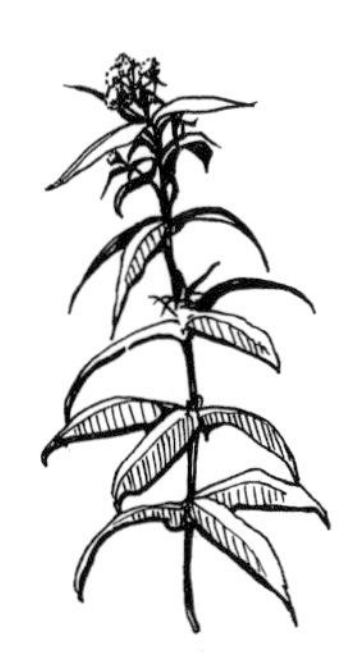

Excellent for 'bone breaking' flu, and also for recurrent febrile conditions and malaria. The patient often complains of unbearable pains in the limbs or the back, sometimes in the muscles, but most typically felt directly in the bones. The pain is often described "as if the bones are broken." No wonder this remedy is also useful to alleviate pains in fractured bones.

AILMENTS AND SYMPTOMS: Unbearable headache in influenza, during or after the fever. Head heavy. High fever preceded by chills and rigor, especially from 7 a.m. to 9 a.m. Restlessness, with pains like *Rhus Tox* yet unlike *Rhus Tox* whose pains are better for movement. The pains of *Eupatorium* are worse from motion. Useful in backache or lumbago with the above characteristics. Great thirst for cold drinks, especially during the chill. May desire cold foods and ice cream. 'Gastric flu' with nausea and vomiting worse during the chills; worse from motion. A raw, painful cough may eventually develop. **Symptoms worsen:** From cold air. Coughing. Sight or smell of food. **Symptoms improve:** After vomiting of bile. From perspiration. Warmth.

EUPHRASIA
(Eyebright)

An important coryza and hay fever medicine.

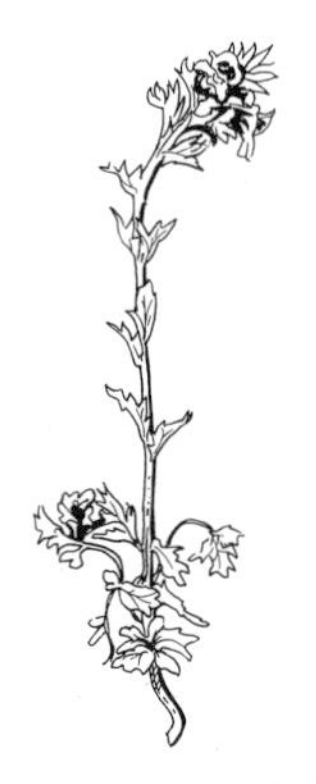

AILMENTS AND SYMPTOMS: Coryza or allergy which is centred especially in the eyes. Bland, non-irritating discharge from the nose, with irritating lachrymation (tears) from the eyes. Pus in the eyes. Eyes burn and smart. Conjunctivitis. Cough with lachrymation. Cartarrhal cough with raw sore larynx. Cough in daytime, better lying down, better in bed at night. Allergic asthma. Hayfever. Allergy. Colds. Whooping cough. First stage of measles, to protect eyes. **Symptoms worsen:** From warm room. **Symptoms improve:** In open air.

FERRUM PHOS
(Iron Phosphate)

A combination of the qualities of *Ferrum* and *Phosphorus*. Assertiveness of *Ferrum* (Iron) combines with the friendly effervescence and excitability of *Phosphorus*. Irritable, loquacious and excitable nature. Restless and nervous. Workaholic: cannot sit still. Quarrelsome and bossy. Need for company. Fear of death, disease, people.

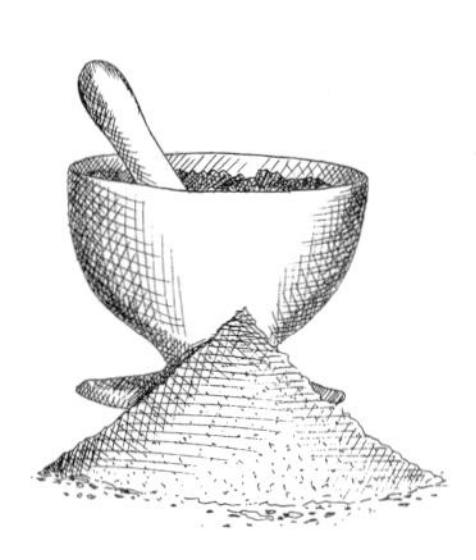

AILMENTS AND SYMPTOMS: A remedy for inflammations of the mucous membranes or joints anywhere in the body. Face flushed, with circumscribed redness of the cheeks. Tendency to inflammations of upper respiratory tract and kidneys. Throat inflammations that result in nephritis. *Ferrum Phos* is an important remedy for initial stage of fevers, inflammations and haemorrhages like *Aconite*. It may be alternated with *Aconite*. Fever during dentition. Nosebleeds - bright, red blood. Burning and rawness in the throat. Dry hacking cough. Violent earache. Rheumatic inflammations of joints. Raynaud's syndrome. **Symptoms worsen:** From cold air. At night. Cold drinks. From suppressed sweat. **Symptoms improve:** With cold applications. Rest.

GELSEMIUM
(Yellow Jasmine)

Complaints that come on after shock: weakness, tremor and collapse. Vacant and dull. Sensitive, delicate people. Old people who are weakened after illness. Delicate and nervous old people with fear of crowds and bustle. Anticipatory fears before examinations or ordeals of any sort that cause feelings of weakness and tremor. Diarrhoea and urge to urinate from anticipation, like *Argentum Nit.* Fear of failure. Fear of going out, of crowds. Agoraphobia. Fear of falling in old people who have weakness, tremor and dizziness.

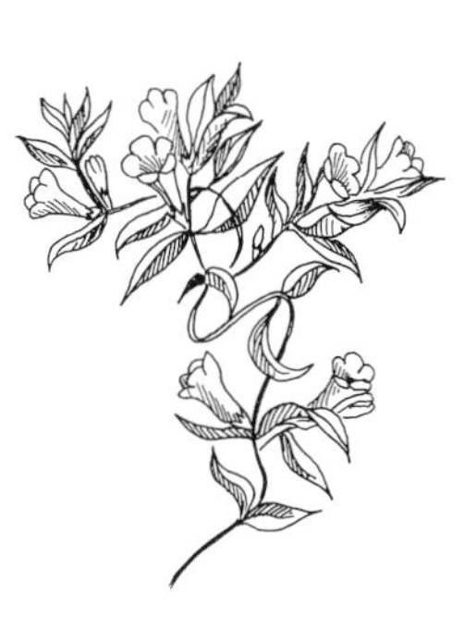

AILMENTS AND SYMPTOMS: Weakness, tremor, and collapse are three key features of *Gelsemium*. Fevers, influenza or nervous states which have these three qualities prominently. It is a leading remedy for shock (*Aconite; Arnica*) and one of the most frequently indicated influenza remedies. Influenza comes on slowly with a stuffy, congested nose and head, headache and scratchy throat. Chills and sneezing, with need to be covered. Weakness, vertigo, tremor, and aching in the muscles develop. Don't want to be disturbed. Want to lie still. Too weak and dizzy to rise. Limpness. Thirstless during fever. Never well since flu. Paralysis after influenza. **Symptoms worsen:** From exertion, mental and physical, or stress. From cold air and changing weather. **Symptoms improve:** After urinating. With warmth. With alcoholic drinks.

GRAPHITES
(Pure Carbon)

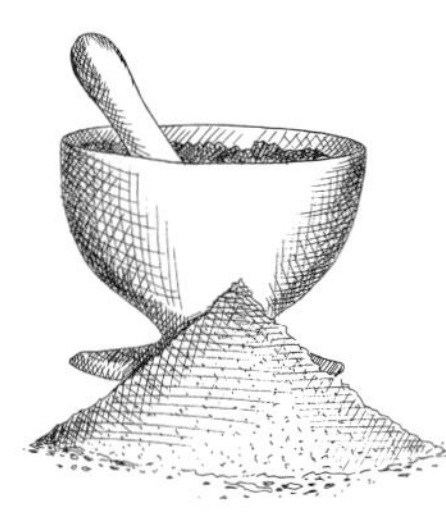

People who are kind, sensitive and have a dislike of quarrels or disharmony. Usually earthy or sensual in some ways, liking music or gardening. Sometimes non-intellectual, manual workers. Often very indecisive. Hesitate over trifles buying a new brand at the supermarket, etc. Depression with pessimism and a feeling of heaviness of mind and body. Feeling of heavy feet. Easily discouraged by setbacks and difficulties. Life seems like a great struggle. Feeling that a disaster will befall them. Worry about the future. Sensitive to music. Timid children.

AILMENTS AND SYMPTOMS: Sluggishness of digestion and of circulation along with poor oxygenation. Tendency to obesity. Hypo-thyroid (*Calc Carb*). Numbness and burning sensations. Pale mucous membranes: lips. Alternative digestive and skin problems. Skin unhealthy, chapped, thickened, coarse, callouses, corns, cracks and fissures. Cracks in feet and hands, behind ears, in corners of mouth, eyes, rectum. Eruptions ooze sticky yellow fluid like honey. Eruptions and fissures in folds, between fingers and toes. Skin eruptions with itching worse from heat of bed like *Sulphur* and *Psorinum*. Scratches till it bleeds. Keloids. Cysts and indurations of skin. Cancerous cysts. Nails brittle. Eyes: blepharitis, eczema of eyelids. Photophobia. Heartburn with flatulence. Constipation with fissures of rectum. Haemorrhoids which are itchy. Nipples sore, cracked. Fibrocystic breasts. Cancer of mammae. Voice hoarse and husky. Often dislike sweet things. Like chicken. **Symptoms worsen:** From cold. During menses. At night. From fats. From suppressing eruptions. **Symptoms improve:** When walking in the open air.

HAMAMELIS

(Witch Hazel)

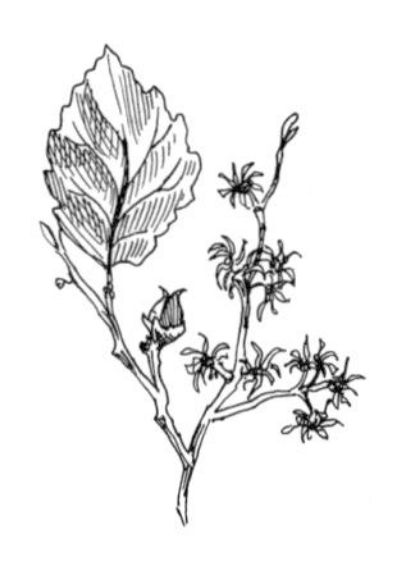

Known for its use in the treatment of varicose veins, *Hamamelis* has a toning and contracting effect on the tissues, particularly the veins.

AILMENTS AND SYMPTOMS: Veins which are hard, knotty, swollen, painful, inflamed, and sensitive. Varicose veins during pregnancy. *Hamamelis* is a powerful styptic: stopping bleeding in haemorrhages from anywhere in the body. It may be alternated with *Arnica* in the treatment of bruises. Black eye - give after *Arnica*, or alternate. Bleeding piles. It is used in many pile ointments. Like *Arnica* it treats a sensation of bruised soreness of the affected parts. It quickly stops nosebleeds or bleeding after dental surgery. It is one of the main remedies for painful inflammation or the veins or phlebitis (*Vipera*).

HEPAR SULPH

(Calcium and Sulphur compounded by heat)

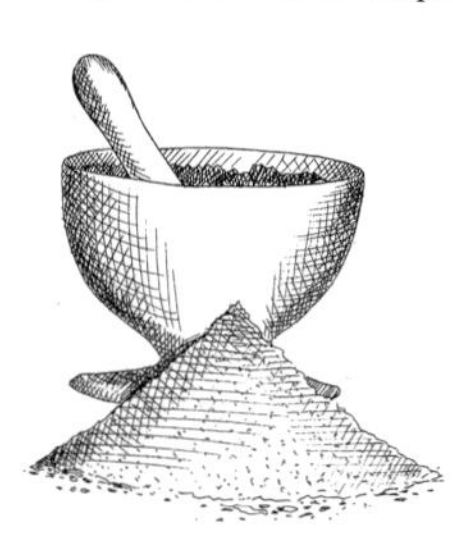

Calcium and *Sulphur* have been heated together to form this compound. The "heat" from the *Sulphur* compound of this remedy and the way it has been made, manifest in angry outbreaks and intense impatience. The *Calcium* component accounts for obstinacy. Morose and touchy adults or children. Very irritable, with outbursts of anger. Could kill with anger. Takes things too personally. Quarrelsome, hard to get along with, nothing pleases him, dislikes persons, places; becomes cross and violent. Irritable or dissatisfied, with self and others. Manic depression. Worries about health. Sensitive to external impressions, pain, noise, cold, draughts.

AILMENTS AND SYMPTOMS: This remedy is known mainly for its effectiveness in relieving colds, flu and rattling coughs, where the conditions worsen at night and from exposure to cold, dry weather, or exposing parts of body to draft. The '*Hepar* constitution' is as vulnerable physically as mentally. Infections easily establish themselves in the form of fever or sepsis, and locally, with abscess formation and suppuration. The person is particularly susceptible to any external influences: weather, noise, light, chemicals and especially cold. These external factors seem to penetrate the patient more easily than any other remedy type. Chilly and aggravated by cold. One of the most cold-sensitive remedies. Intolerant of becoming cold. Generally worse uncovering a hand or foot, or touching a cold surface. Intolerant to draughts, and especially to cold dry winds. Earache comes on from draughts or wind. Sore throat with pains like splinters. Suppurating tonsils. Croup. Rattling cough, worse on waking and after midnight. Offensive discharges. Infected, yellow discharges from nose, eyes, or lungs. Sticking pains. Abscesses or boils which are very painful to touch. Acne. Face reddish or blue-red colour. **Symptoms worsen:** From cold, dry air. Cold weather. Winter. Cold draughts. Exposing body to cold. Noise. Lying on painful part. Night. **Symptoms improve:** With heat, and warm wraps. Warm wraps to head. Warm, moist weather.

HYPERICUM

(St. John's Wort)

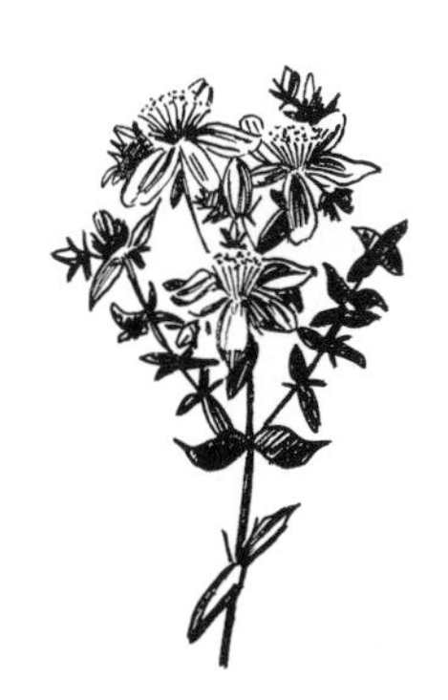

One of the important remedies for injury, especially nerve-rich areas of the body. It quickly relieves the pains of injury to fingers, toes, nails and spine.

AILMENTS AND SYMPTOMS: Pain in the coccyx after a fall or after childbirth. Neuritis arising after injury with tingling, burning and numbness. Relieves pain after operations. Should be alternated with *Arnica* after to relieve pains and bruising after dental surgery. The pains of *Hypericum* are often sharp and shooting. Where *Calendula* promotes healing of superficial abrasions, *Hypericum* is preferable for deep wounds. If applied as a tincture to deep wounds and punctures with pointed instruments, it prevents anaerobic infection including tetanus. Needle injuries with continued nerve pains. Phantom limb pain. Painful scars. Convulsions due to trauma of the head or spine. Concussion. Depression with feelings of melancholy and irritability. **Symptoms worsen:** After injury or surgery. Jarring. Concussion; of spine, coccyx. Shock. Bruises. Exertion. Touch. Change of weather. Fog. Cold, damp. Motion. After forceps delivery, as a complication of injury. **Symptoms improve:** Lying on face. Bending back. Rubbing.

IPECAC

(Ipecacuana root)

Known for its use in asthmatic rattling coughs and gastric derangements with nausea, vomiting and diarrhoea.

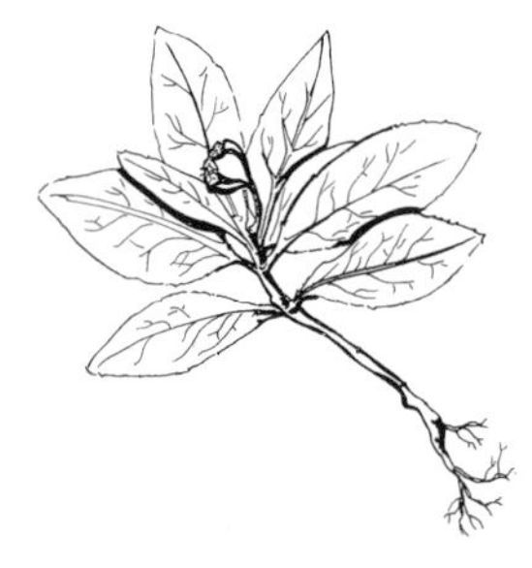

AILMENTS AND SYMPTOMS: Persistent nausea, which is not relieved by vomiting. Profuse salivation. The tongue is usually clean. Catarrhal conditions of the stomach: may vomit mucus. Gastric upsets from rich pastry, candy, ice cream like *Pulsatilla*, but unlike *Pulsatilla*, nausea continues after vomiting. Nausea of pregnancy which is not relieved by vomiting. Stomach feels relaxed as if hanging down. Diarrhoea in which the stool appears to be fermented like yeast, or green as grass, or watery, or is slimy and dysenteric, with more or less blood. Autumn dysentery. Pale face with dark rings about the eyes. Asthma with oppressed breathing. Wheezing and rattling without expectoration. Vomits with cough. Whooping cough: child loses his breath, turns pale, stiff and blue in the face; suffocating cough with gagging and vomiting of mucous. There may be bleeding from nose or mouth. Complaints have spasmodic, rigid and convulsive character. Thirstlessness. Antidote to the morphine/heroine habit. **Symptoms worsen:** From warmth. Dampness. Overeating rich foods and pastry. Cold water may trigger cough. **Symptoms improve:** With rest. Pressure. Cold drinks.

IGNATIA

(St. Ignatius' Bean)

A much used remedy for emotional shock, grief and disappointment. Grief after loss of someone close. Grief which may be internalised and unexpressed. Cry alone (*Nat Mur*). Idealistic, romantic and ambitious people. Idealise relationships, career,

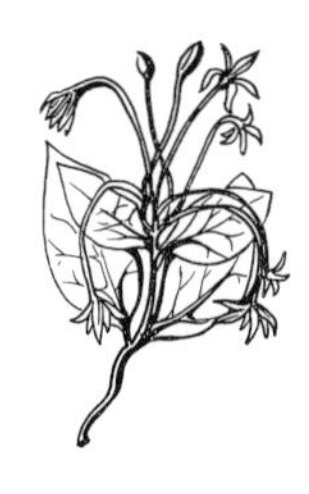

future projects etc. and become disappointed when reality fails to match up. Want to be a perfect mother, or perfect actress. Guilt and remorse over past failures. Religious fanaticism. Expressive children and adults. Theatrical and dramatic. Often interested in theatre, literature or art. Creative bent. Desire for excellence in literature or ballet. Cultural interests. Sensitive to injustice. Easily offended. Sensitive teenagers. Moods changeable and unpredictable. Sudden hysterical outbursts. Fear of failure and rejection. Fear of birds.

AILMENTS AND SYMPTOMS: *Ignatia* contains strychnine like *Nux Vom*. This substance accounts for the twitches, spasms and cramps that characterize the remedy. Changeable symptoms. Spasmodic symptoms. Neuralgias. Spasms of facial muscles. Tension in the jaws. Frequent sighing is common. Headaches after grief or disappointment. Schoolgirl headaches (*Pulsatilla; Calc Carb*). Headaches like a nail being driven into the temple. Spasm of larynx or oesophagus with a feeling of a 'lump' and choking sensation. Cramping pains in the abdomen after emotions (*Colocynth; Nux Vom*; all the *Magnesias*). Constipation. Sneezing attacks. Spasmodic cough. Constriction of chest. Loss of voice. Yawning and sighing. Very sensitive to tobacco smoke. (*Nux Vom; Nat Mur; Staphysagria*). Paralytic symptoms come on after grief or hurt. Tremors and spasms of muscles. Trembling hands. Spasm of back or neck. Premenstrual tension, with oversensitive reactions and emotional outbursts. **Symptoms worsen:** From emotions, grief or hurt. Fright or shock. Tobacco. Yawning. Stooping, walking, standing. **Symptoms improve:** With change of position. Applying pressure. Urination. If alone. Deep breathing. Eating.

KALI BICH

(Potassium Bichromate)

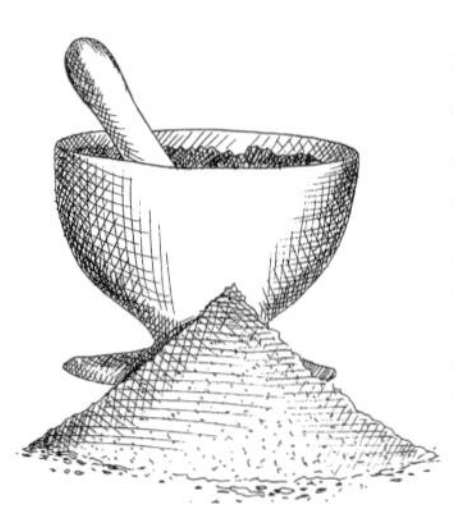

This remedy is known for painful sinusitis and chronic post- nasal drip. All the *Kali* remedies, particularly *Kali Carb* are conservative and correct. Things are black or white. Live by the book. Like to make the right impression. Pedantic detail when describing anything. Analytical, logical mind. Helpful to others. May be unsociable, preferring company of family or like-minded people. Shy. Dislike crowds. Fastidious: desire for symmetry.

AILMENTS AND SYMPTOMS: Pains in small spots. Catarrh or discharge from any mucous membranes which are gelatinous, slimy, sticky and stringy. Sinusitis with sinus headaches. Blurred vision before headaches. Pain over a small area on forehead or occipital. Mucus sticks in the larynx. Catarrhal laryngitis (*Ferr Phos; Hepar Sulph; Mercurius*). Croup or hoarse cough with sticky mucous in the larynx and trachea. Digestive and bowel complaints. Punched out ulcers in the mouth and stomach. Mucous colitis. Stitching pains anywhere. Wandering symptoms, e.g. arthritis. **Symptoms worsen:** From beer, wine, milk products. From heat. During spring and autumn. **Symptoms improve:** With pressure. During motion.

KALI MUR

(Potassium Chloride)

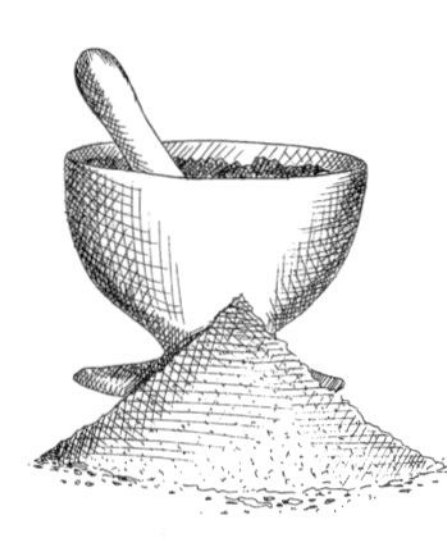

Conservative, conscientious and anxious. Sympathetic and caring about family. Emotionally sensitive, easily hurt and hysterical. Need for a caring approach from others. Weakness after emotions. Family types. Hate aggression. Sensitive children who are easily hurt. Anxiety which may be felt in the abdomen.

AILMENTS AND SYMPTOMS: Affections of muscles, mucous membranes, and liver. Weakness. Pains in muscles, joints and back. Fibrositis. Arthritis. Myalgic encephalo-myelitis. Many foods disagree. Mucus secretions from mucous membranes are white, like egg albumin (*Nat Mur*), sometimes yellow. Colds, catarrhs, sinusitis, catarrhal deafness. Post nasal drip. Glue ear. Oral or vaginal thrush. White vaginal discharge. Sterility. Liver and digestion disturbed. Fullness after eating. Indigestion from fat or rich foods. Jaundice. Diarrhoea with slimy stools. Swelling of glands. Measles. Nephritis. High cholesterol. Tendency to thrombosis: phlegmasia alba dolens. Phlebitis. Embolism. White patches on skin. Eczema with white flakey scales. Water retention in extremities. **Symptoms worsen:** At night. From open air and draughts. After eating, fats and rich foods. From cold, bathing. **Symptoms improve:** Cold drinks. Rubbing.

KALI PHOS

(Potassium Phosphate)

Conservative people who identify with a particular group, club or sect. Need for support from friends and associates. Startle

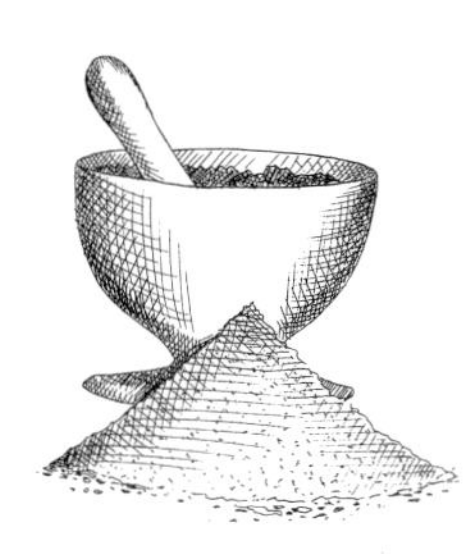

easily. Ailments come on from shock, stress or worry. Nervous exhaustion or depression after tiring mental work. Exam nerves (fear of exams). Worries too much about business or about others. Anxiety about relationships. Worries about health. Imagine disease. Hypochondriac. Fear of being alone, of the dark, of disease, death, evil; of people. Fear of noise. Startles easily. Aversion to certain people. Whining, fretful children. Crying and screaming.

AILMENTS AND SYMPTOMS: Weakness. Colds with white discharge. The first stage of sinusitis and post nasal drip (*Kali Sulph* or *Kali Bich* for the later stage). Fibrositis. Pain and tension in shoulders. Ill effects from any bodily or mental stress, worries, grief or vexation. Paralysis after mental stress. Nervous exhaustion. Headaches after mental exertion. Vertigo. Chronic fatigue. Headaches from mental strain. Nervous heart. Palpitations and asthma. Diarrhoea from shock or from nerves. **Symptoms worsen:** From worry, mental or physical exertion, stress. **Symptoms improve:** With rest, warmth and bathing.

KALI SULPH

(Potassium Sulphate)

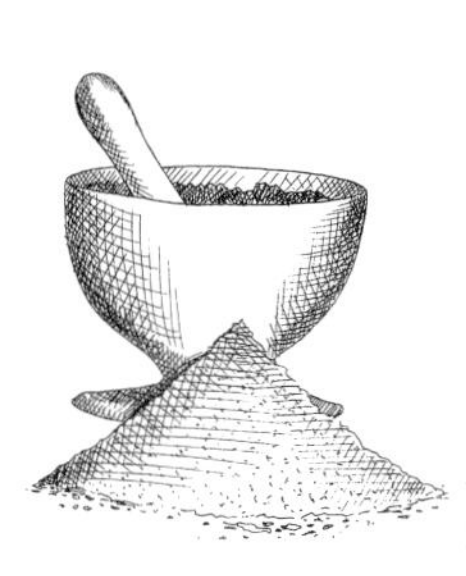

Kali Sulph is a tissue salt which is known for relieving ailments with yellow discharges. Depression - cannot motivate themselves. Tired, critical, irritable, impatient moods. Restless. Aversion to work. Loss of self-confidence. Anxiety felt in the abdomen or chest. Worries about family. Confusion and difficulty concentrating. Pedantic: give a detailed account of illness. Dogmatic - think they know it all. Sceptical and opinionated.

AILMENTS AND SYMPTOMS: Similar to *Pulsatilla* but there is thirst. Mucous membranes produce deep yellow, sticky discharges. Allergic rhinitis. Sinusitis. Eustachian deafness (*Kali Mur*). Rattling cough with yellow expectoration and weakness. Asthma. Jaundice. Weak digestion with heartburn. Diarrhoea with yellow stools. Wandering arthritic pains. Scaling, chapping skin, and eruptions with burning and itching. Eruptions with yellow discharge. Urethral or vaginal discharges: yellow and offensive. **Symptoms worsen:** From warmth, noise, evening. **Symptoms improve:** Cold. Fresh air. Walking. Fasting.

LACHESIS

(Bushmaster Viper - venom)

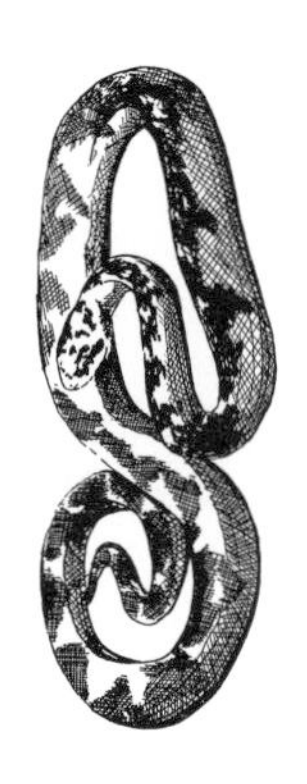

Excitable and intense people who are often talkative. Not good listeners. Too busy projecting themselves. Passionate and animated. Often very creative: writers or artists. Intensity in relationships and jealousy drive people away. Workaholics. Untidy and often late for appointments like *Sulphur*. Intense negative feelings if crossed. Revengeful. Distrust of others. Paranoid jealousy. Often very sexual. Interest in philosophy (*Lycopodium*) and religion. Religious fanaticism. Children who are jealous and talkative. Attention seeking. Asthma from sibling jealousy. Excitable children; seek stimulation (*Phosphorus*). Usually confident and outgoing. Anxiety attacks with palpitations on lying down to go to sleep or on waking in morning. Claustrophobia. Fear of snakes, closed places, robbers, heart disease, cancer, thunderstorms.

AILMENTS OR SYMPTOMS: Left sided symptoms, dislike or worsening from heat, and dislike of tight clothes or wraps; are the main features that distinguish *Lachesis*. Left sided symptoms: throat pains, otitis, headaches and pains. Constricted or tight feeling. Pains over the left side of the chest, Left ovary pains. Clotted menses. Premenstrual tension. Menopausal flushes. Circulatory symptoms with flushes or aggravation from heat. Palpitations. Pulsations. Blueness of parts: cheeks, fingers, feet, nose and lips. Netted veins on cheeks. Brown circles under eyes. Eyed may protrude with a staring look. Goitre. Soft cauliflower moles or red moles (*Thuja*) on the skin. Wear loose fitting clothes: particularly around neck. Sensitivity of skin to touch. Skin eruptions with scaling, worse from heat. Septic states: abscesses and boils. Glandular fever. Mouth ulcers. Tired at noon or 2 p.m. Desire for pasta, shellfish and coffee. **Symptoms worsen:** While falling asleep, after sleep or on waking. From hot or stuffy places. Touch or pressure. Tight clothing. Before menses or during menopause. In foggy weather. **Symptoms improve:** In open air. From discharges: e.g. once menses starts. Cold applications. Movement.

LEDUM

(Marsh Tea/Wild Rosemary)

Well known as a remedy for punctured wounds produced by

sharp, pointed instruments, particularly if the wound is cold. It prevents tetanus.

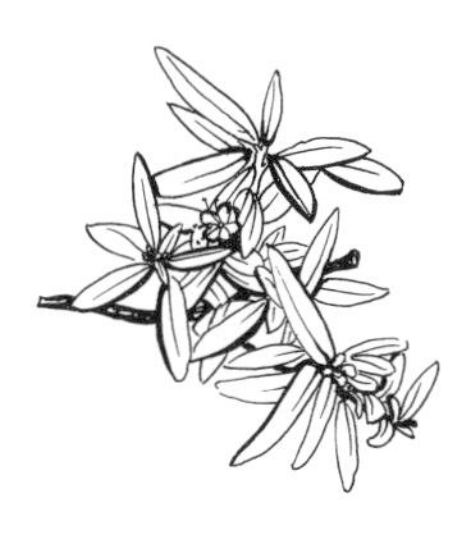

AILMENTS AND SYMPTOMS: Itchy, irritating bites of insects, fleas, mosquitoes, spiders. It may be applied as a lotion and taken internally. Nettle rash worse in the heat of the bed (*Pulsatilla*). Gout and rheumatism where pains begin in the feet and extend to the body. Gouty swellings and nodes around the joints (*Colchicum*). Pale, puffy swellings which are inflamed, may become purple. Pains in the joints are worse from the heat of the bed, and better from cold applications. Worse from motion. Pains in soles of feet, ankles and knees. Pains may affect small joints of hands and feet. Removes bruises and follows *Arnica* well to remove bruises of the face or around the eye after blows or surgery. Useful in bruises that remain a long time. Emotionally, the person needing *Ledum* may be angry and discontented. Aversion to friends. Hatred. **Symptoms worsen:** From warmth of covers. Motion. Injuries. Night. From wine. **Symptoms improve:** With cold bathing, cold air. Rest.

LYCOPODIUM
(Club Moss)

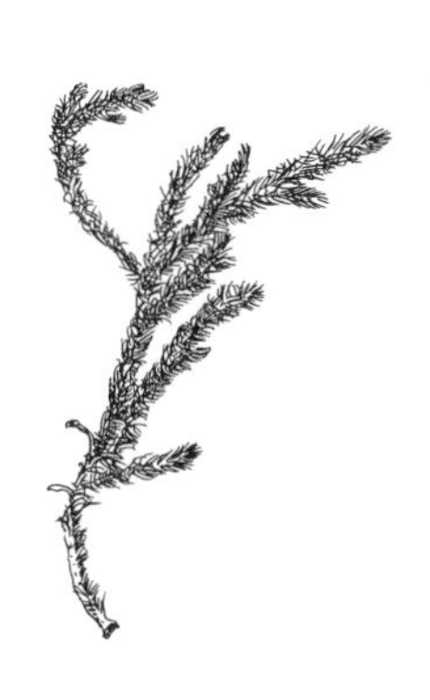

Competitive and ambitious people (*Lachesis* and *Nux Vom*) who are driven to succeed by an underlying sense of inadequacy. Marked lack of confidence. Project a front of confidence. Joke a lot. May take classes in public speaking. May exaggerate or brag. Successful type. Overconcerned about status. Ingratiating and charming toward authorities. Arrogant and abusive to weaker mortals: subordinates, wife and children. Dislike being judged. Suffer from anticipation nerves before public performance, yet may get to like to perform. Hypochondriacal. Imagine disease. Bouts of depression with desire to be left alone. Children lack confidence with strangers or in new situations and may fear speaking out in class. Children with dyslexia who lack confidence and dislike detailed intellectual work. Fears of cancer, being alone, commitment, public speaking. Agoraphobia. Philosophic. Often become professionals - teachers, priests, lawyers. May become actors. Deep need to achieve something.

AILMENTS AND SYMPTOMS: Frown marks on the forehead are a common physical feature of this remedy. It is a well known remedy for liverishness with irritability, bloating, gas and a tendency to constipation or haemorrhoids. Gas and distension worse from raw vegetables, onions, and cabbage family. Constipation and haemorrhoids. Liver underfunction. Hepatitis. Inflammation of gall bladder (Cholecystitis). Right-sided pains generally. Pharyngitis or tonsillitis often right-sided or begins on the right, improved with warm or cold drinks. Right sided pneumonia. Kidney stone colic (*Colocynthis*), right side, may have reddish sand in the urine. Right-sided varicosities. Skin eruptions, palmar eruptions, psoriasis. Weariness and irritability, worse between 4 p.m. to 8 p.m. Impotence and premature ejaculation. Tumours and polyps of bowel. Desires sweet things, and warm drinks - tea or coffee. **Symptoms worsen:** From pressure of clothing. Heat. On waking. Wind. Eating; even a little. Oysters and cabbage. **Symptoms improve:** With warm drinks. Cold applications. Motion. Passing wind. Urinating.

MAG PHOS

(Magnesium Phosphate)

Sociable, open, friendly and warm people. Care about others. Mediate and help to solve disputes. Like all the *Magnesiums* they are very sensitive to disharmony. Protect the underdog (*Causticum*). Irritable and mentally fagged. Like to keep busy and find it difficult to relax. Tend to be scatty; rushing about fruitlessly. Ambitious. Dislike seeing violence or blood. Avoid gory movies.

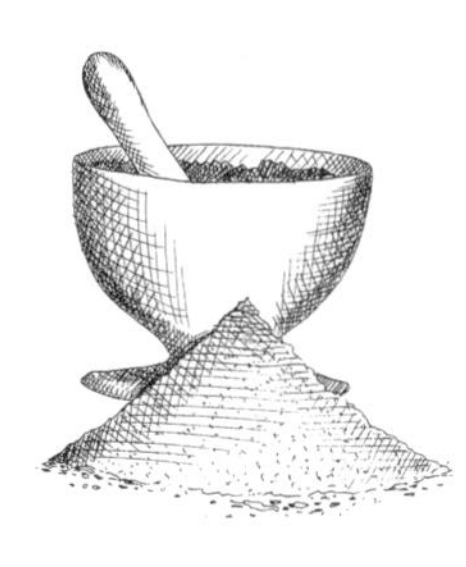

AILMENTS AND SYMPTOMS: Neuralgias or pains which improve with warmth. Neuralgic pains in the face or anywhere. Brain fag. Headache after mental activity. Cramps in limbs and abdomen. Torticollis. Hiccoughs. Angina. Pains during teething. General pain reliever. **Symptoms worsen:** Cold air. Drafts. Touch. Night. **Symptoms improve:** Warmth. Pressure. Doubling up. Rubbing.

MERCURIUS

(Mercury)

Mercury vaporises easily and scatters into thousands of pieces if dropped. It amalgamates well with other metals. Poisoning causes

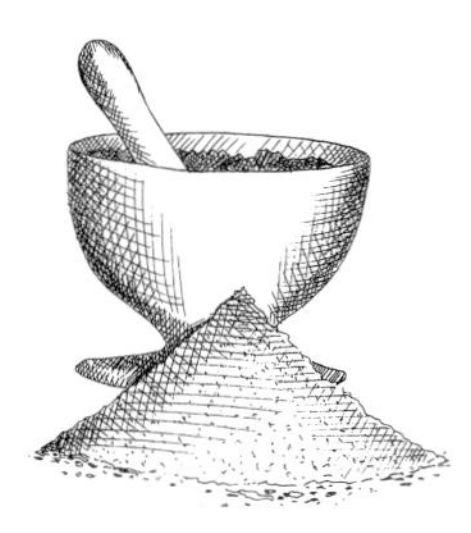

much salivation, ulceration of membranes, easy sweating, nervous tremor and mental disturbances. Bloody diarrhoea and nephritis with bloody urine occurs. These are the main symptoms for which *Mercurius* is therapeutic. Mercury has mental characteristics of scattered, uncertain behaviour and speech. Feel fragile and need a stable environment. Often childlike or immature in some way. They sometimes stay with parents even as adults. They may have an immature attitude to work, lacking ambition. They don't feel they are fully in command of their lives or themselves. Scattered and impulsive approach to things. Hasty rapid speech. Stammering. Scatty children with attention problems. Very intelligent when they concentrate.

AILMENTS AND SYMPTOMS: Great variety of symptoms. Salivation especially at night in sleep. Sensitive to heat or cold, like a mercury thermometer. Metallic taste in mouth. Strong halitosis. Perspiration all over their bodies, which may be offensive. Tongue swollen with imprint of teeth. Tongue coated white or yellow; looks wet. Dry mouth with thirst. Dry lips. Discharges from mucous membrane: nose, throat, vagina or rectum; tends to be offensive. Sinusitis. Vaginitis. Stomatitis. Thrush. Ulcers anywhere, on tongue, mouth, and throat. Swollen glands anywhere on the body. Glandular fever. Recurrent tonsillitis with suppurating, rotten tonsils. Breath offensive. Recurring otitis media with 'glue ear'. Green, thick nasal discharge or sputum from throat. Herpes around mouth or genitals. Moist eruptions with foul discharge. Ulcerative colitis. Desires bread and butter intensely. Dislikes sweets (*Graphites*, *Phosphorus*). **Symptoms worsen:** At night. From heat and cold, and from changes of temperature. From perspiration. In open air, wet weather. From stress, over-work, confusion, chaos. **Symptoms improve:** In quiet, even environment, and in warm dry weather.

NAT MUR

(Common Table Salt)

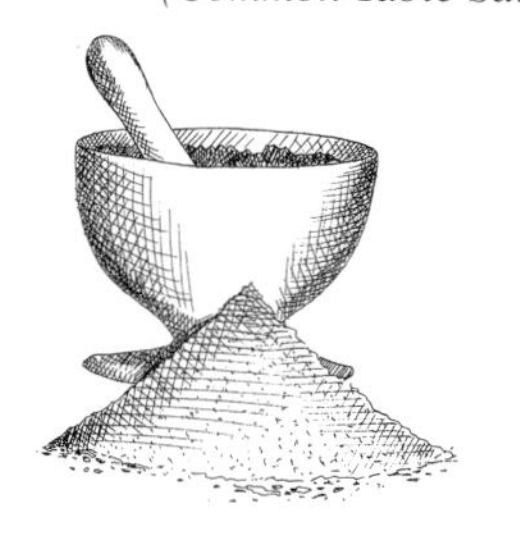

'Salt of the earth' type of people. Self-contained, reserved and modest people who are good listeners but never complain. Children and adults who are sympathetic and caring for others, but don't like talking about their own problems. Responsible and considerate to others. Often counsellors or social workers. Givers more than receivers. Find it difficult to ask for help. Long-term effects of grief and internalised hurt. Chronic internalised grief (acute grief *Ignatia*). Like their own company. Keep people at a distance through fear of being hurt. Serious. Perfectionist. Like routine. Have a set way of doing things. Children reserved, serious, responsible, take care of parents or of other children. Like reading and spending time by themselves. Awkward, shy and sensitive teenagers. Fear of closed places, robbers, spiders, germs, heights and failure.

AILMENTS AND SYMPTOMS: Imagine the effects of salt: dryness of mucosa, giving rise to thirst and constipation. Dryness of skin, dandruff, herpes around lips, oedema, cracks in middle of lower lip and corners of mouth, contractions of muscles, cramps, dryness of synovial fluid therefore cracking of joints. Paralysis, with numbness. Tremors. Headaches from the sun, start forenoon. Anaemia. Palpitations. Weakness. Myalgic encephalo-myelitis. Thrush: vaginal and oral. Mapped tongue. Acne in teenagers or adults. Greasy hair and skin which may be pale. Hay fever. Urticaria or hives (*Apis*; *Pulsatilla, Rhus Tox*). Premenstrual tension. Menses scanty or absent. Amenorrhoea after grief (*Ignatia*). Sterility in closed people. Constipation from unexpressed feelings. Cold hands and feet. Hangnails. Bites fingernails. Desires salty foods, bread and soup. Dislikes fats. **Symptoms worsen:** From 9 a.m. to 11 a.m. From the heat of the sun. Emotions. Sympathy. Puberty. Touch. **Symptoms improve:** In open air. Cool bathing. Sweating. Rest. Going without regular meals.

NAT PHOS

(Sodium Phosphate)

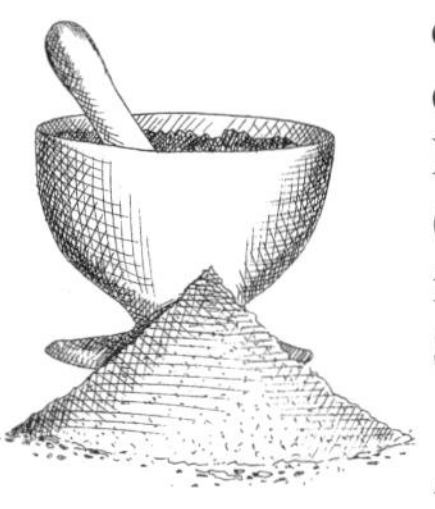

The most open and sociable of the *Natrums*. The *Phosphorus* component creates a need for company, yet a tendency to become withdrawn and find it difficult to become close. Worry. Nervous, startle easily. Scattered. Difficulty with concentration (learning disorders). Fearful. Vivid imagination: imagines clothing on chair at night to be a burglar. Imagines hearing footsteps. Sensitive to music.

AILMENTS AND SYMPTOMS: Discharges from eyes, nose, and vagina tend to be thick and yellow. Sinusitis. Tongue coated yellow at base. Sour belching and flatulence. Dryness of mucous membranes. Acid state of blood resulting in arthritic pains, cracking of joints, vaginal or oral thrush, itching of nose and itching of rectum. Worms. Candida. Water retention. Nervous exhaustion. Palpitations after emotions. Trembling, numbness, cold extremities, and contractions of muscles: cramps. **Symptoms worsen:** From sugar or sweets. Milk. Mental exertion. Thunderstorm. Gas light. Coitus. Walking upstairs. Bitter foods. Fatty foods. **Symptoms improve:** Cold. Avoiding sweet things.

NAT SULPH

(Sodium Sulphate)

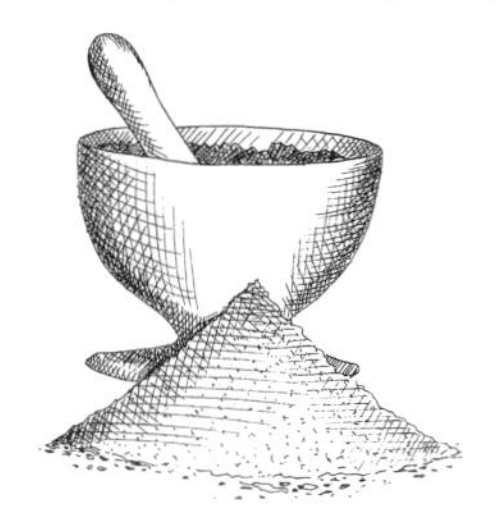

Often very focused people, achievers, successful businessmen. Self-centred, impatient and lazy at times. Less considerate and well mannered than *Nat Mur.* Workaholics. Withdrawn, irritable and morose. Averse to company. Cannot get close to partner. Depression with suicidal thoughts. Manic depressive. Depression after head injury. Depression becomes worse from listening to music. Anxiety attacks. Ailments from wounded honour. Fears of crowds, narrow places, misfortune and suicide.

AILMENTS AND SYMPTOMS: Confusion, depression or epilepsy after head injury. Liverishness with much flatulence. Pain and discomfort over the liver. Early morning diarrhoea. Sinusitis, discharges (gonorrhoea and leucorrhoea). Asthma or bronchitis worse from damp weather, worse early morning. Hangnails. **Symptoms worsen:** During damp weather; night air. In damp rooms or cellars. Injuries; to head. Lifting. Music. Late evening. Vegetables, fruits. Cold food and drinks. Lying long in one position. **Symptoms improve:** In open air. Lying on back.

NUX VOMICA

(Poison Nut)

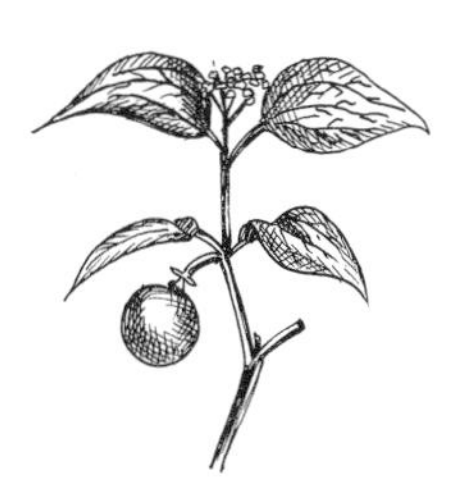

The '*Nux Vomica* type' tends to be an 'A type': driving and ambitious. They are competitive and efficient. Like method and order, and become angry about inefficiency or if things are not in their correct place. Domineering personalities. Good leaders. Set high standards. Hate injustice. Take on too much. Worry about money. Bouts of violent anger if under stress. Insomnia, with early waking: 3 a.m. to 5 a.m. Wake from the smallest sound. Sensitive to external impressions: noise, light, odours and disorder. Children are fastidious and competitive. Goal oriented. Poor losers. Concerned about fairness. Craving for stimulants (especially coffee and alcohol). Needs coffee to work, and alcohol to sleep.

AILMENTS AND SYMPTOMS: Known for its positive effects on digestive problems of all sorts, particularly those that arise from overindulgence in rich foods and alcohol. Ailments from overindulgence; from working too hard and playing too hard. Digestive symptoms are usually prominent. Symptoms usually come on from stress. Cramping pains and spasms anywhere in the body. Intestinal spasms, oesophageal spasms (Hiatus Hernia), urethral spasms (Stricture), gall duct spasm (Cholecystitis) etc. Cramps in legs or feet at night in bed. Cramping, colic pains in the abdomen. Constipation. Diarrhoea after eating. Heartburn and indigestion worse after eating rich or spicy foods. Stomach ulcers. Hepatitis with pains over the liver. Crohn's disease. Haemorrhoids better from warmth and passing stool. Ineffectual urging to stool or to urinate (Cystitis). Hayfever and sneezing with itching of the tubes. Right-sided headaches, with spasm and tension in the neck. Neck and back spasms. Desires fats, spices, highly seasoned foods, rich foods, alcohol, whisky and wine. Aversion to spices and to bland or tasteless foods. **Symptoms worsen:** In early morning. Cold; open air (dry). Draughts. Uncovering. From high living. Coffee. Liquor, drugs, purgatives, overeating. Sedentary habits. Mental exertion and stress. After anger. From disturbed sleep. From noise; odours; touch and pressure. Wounded honour. Mental shock. **Symptoms improve:** Naps. Resting. Warmth. Hot drinks. Milk. Fats. Moist air. Lying on side.

PHOSPHORUS

(Phosphorus)

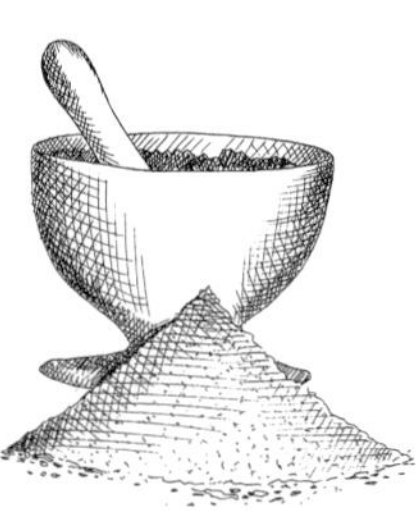

Think of '*Phosphorescence*' in the sea, it conveys an idea of the bright, sparkling character of *Phosophorus*. The word that aptly describes *Phosophorus* types is 'effervescent'. They sparkle with enthusiasm and affability. They may flush up when excited. They are friendly and communicative even with strangers. They have quick minds and are often good with words, intelligent and quick thinking. They are sociable, sympathetic to others and very affectionate, particularly the children. The child is chatty (*Lachesis*) and curious, asking questions about many things. Problems with attention or concentration in both adults and children. Diffusion of mind. Nervous and scattered. Their overactive imaginations create worries. Worry a lot and imagine disasters. Fear of being alone, disease, for others, dark, thunderstorms.

AILMENTS AND SYMPTOMS: Nervous complaints. Nervous exhaustion after stress. Startle easily from noise. Children that grow fast. Nosebleeds, gums bleed, easy bruising. Heavy menses. Tall, thin, hungry. Feel faint and trembling if they miss a meal. Burning pains anywhere. Burning in chest during cough. Burning in stomach. Tendency to get colds which go to chest and cause pneumonia. Nausea and vomiting, with vomiting of food once it warms up in the stomach. Fibroids cause heavy bleeding. Ovarian cysts often worse on the left. Palpitations when lying on the left side (*Lachesis*). Dizziness in old people. Multiple sclerosis. Desire of salt, spicy, bananas, ice cream, chocolate, meat, fish, cold milk, carbonated drinks. Averse to shellfish, fish, eggs, fruit, meat. **Symptoms worsen:** From lying on painful side, or on left side. From excitement or emotions. Odours. Light. Cold. Open air. Puberty. Salt. Changing weather; before thunderstorms. **Symptoms improve:** With rest and sleep. Cold; food, water, washing face with cold water. Massage.

PHYTOLACCA

(Poke Root)

Known as 'vegetable mercury' *Phytolacca* is a glandular remedy, having an affinity particularly for tonsils and breasts. It also benefits ligaments and joints.

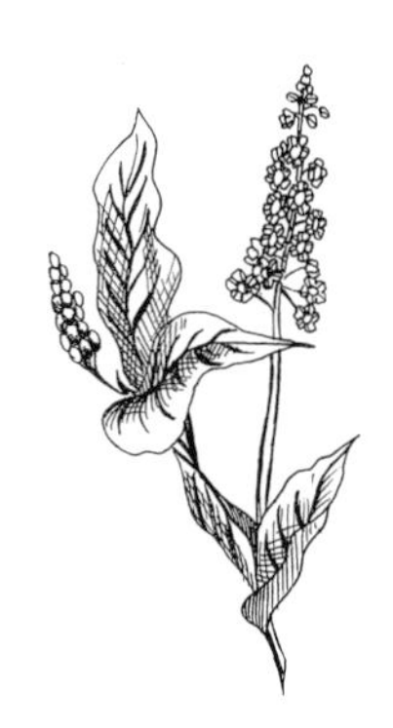

AILMENTS AND SYMPTOMS: Tonsillitis, recurrent or acute. Dark red or blueish-red throat or tonsils with white spots, worse right side; worse from warm drinks, better from cold drinks. Pain extends to the ear on swallowing. Post-nasal drip and sinusitis with a tough, stringy discharge, difficult to detach. Swollen, hard glands. Mumps. Breast stony hard, heavy, swollen or tender. The swelling may appear purple. Breast pains are worse during nursing, spreading over the whole body. Cracked nipples. Hard nodules in breasts; and enlarged auxiliary glands. Chronic discharge from nipples. Sore all over; worse on eyeballs, breasts, kidneys, neck, shoulders, back, forearms and below knees. Fibrositis. Wandering pains come and go; shooting and lanciating, like electric shocks. Rheumatic affections after tonsillitis. Rheumatic swellings hard, tender and intensely hot. Restlessness with desire for motion and worse in cold, damp weather like *Rhus Tox*; but motion aggravates like *Bryonia*. Useful where both *Rhus Tox* and *Bryonia* seem indicated but do not work. Dentition may be delayed or difficult with the child biting teeth together or clenching. **Symptoms worsen:** From becoming wet. During rain. Damp cold weather. Night. Motion. Right side. **Symptoms improve:** With warmth and dry weather. Rest.

PULSATILLA

(Windflower)

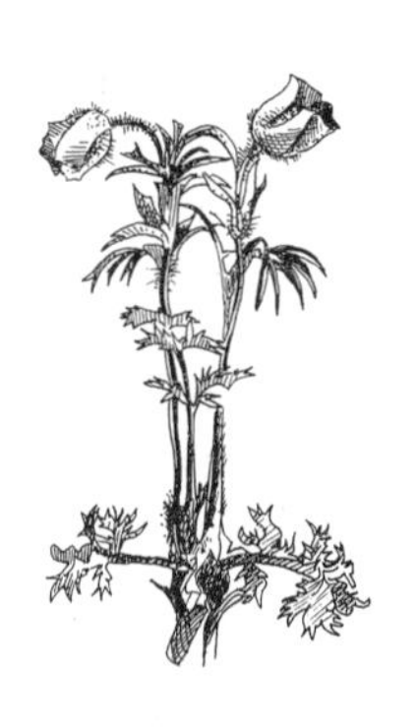

As the name suggests this flower likes wind and fresh air - growing in social groups on hillsides. *Pulsatilla* is famous for disliking heat and stuffiness, and being a window-opener. *Pulsatilla* characters are endearing, affectionate, charming, sweet and sensitive. Their mild manner elicits a 'protective response' from those who encounter them. They like to please others and fear confrontations. They are dependent on others, having a fear of rejection or solitude. Like sympathy if upset or weepy. Sometimes childlike. They easily become moody and tearful particularly before menses. Depression and anxiety. Emotional insecurity. May become fanatically religious. Affectionate, clingy and tearful children. Boys or men who cry easily. Fear of men (in little girls), being alone, heights, poverty, closed places, being attacked. Often blonde, red or blueish face, soft features. Flush easily. Veins may be prominent.

AILMENTS AND SYMPTOMS: Headaches worse from heat. Colds or conjunctivitis with yellow/green discharge. Cough worse on lying down at night, worse in a warm room, and better walking in open air. Loose cough. Digestive disorders, liver disorders with intolerance of rich foods, diverticulitis, gas. Asthma worse from stuffy rooms, and emotions. Otitis media is common in *Pulsatilla* children. Menstrual problems of all kinds: amenorrhoea, dysmenorrhoea, irregularity. Premenstrual tension with sore breasts and tearfulness. Thrush with yellow discharge. Cystitis. Conjunctivitis. Arthritis. Prostatitis. Sluggish circulation with varices and swelling of lower limbs in heat. Bloating and discomfort in the abdomen. Bouts of nausea, worse from rich foods, fats, and cream. Pastry and eggs may aggravate. Often, but not always thirstless. Like to eat fruit and salads. Dislike heavy, starchy foods. **Symptoms worsen:** In evenings and on waking. Heat and warm, stuffy rooms. Lying in bed. During rest. Fats or rich foods. Tight clothing. **Symptoms improve:** With walking in open air. Fresh air. Cool weather. Uncovering. Gentle motion.

RHUS TOX
(Poison Ivy)

The most well known remedy for arthritis and back pains. Tense individuals who start off conversation awkwardly then gain confidence and become talkative. May wake with anxiety at night. Suspicious imaginings about others. Sometimes superstitious.

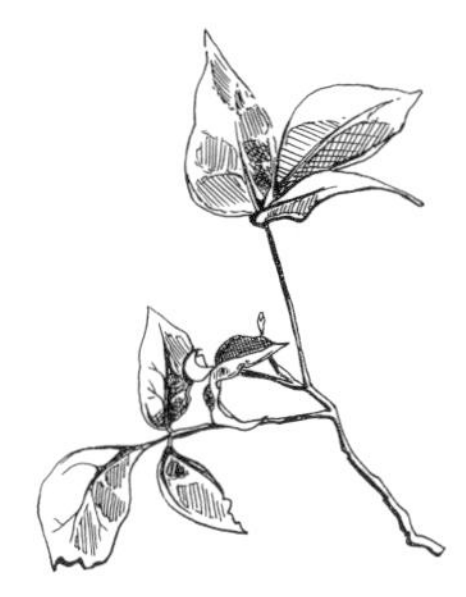

AILMENTS AND SYMPTOMS: Tongue coated with red tip. Arthritic pains worse from damp and cold and better from heat or warm weather (the opposite to *Bryonia*). Pains and stiffness in joints which are worse during rest, and on initial motion and better from continued motion. Hot bathing eases pains. Red triangle on tip of white coated tongue. Sore spots on tongue. Back pains, cervical pains with stiffness worse on rising. Needs to get up and move around. Muscles bound up in neck. Lumbago and sciatica worse from sitting still for long periods. Eruptions on genitalia especially thigh next to groin. Herpes about lips or around genitals. Vesicular eruptions: shingles. Eczema of the hands with burning and itching vesicular eruption. Erythema nodosum. Chicken pox (most important remedy). Influenza with chills, pains and stiffness in the back and joints. Restless legs at night in bed. Desires milk, sweets. Averse to meat. **Symptoms worsen:** During rest. On waking in the morning. Midnight. During cold and/or damp weather (*Dulcamara*). Sitting. From strain or excessive exertion (gentle motion improves). **Symptoms improve:** With warmth and warm bathing. With gentle motion. In warm, dry weather.

RUTA GRAV
(Rue/Bitterwort)

This remedy is indicated in case of strains, bruises and other mechanical injuries of the bones and periosteum.

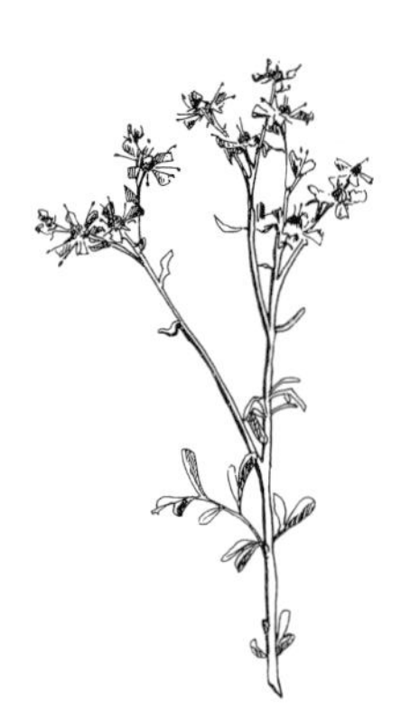

AILMENTS AND SYMPTOMS: Bruised pain in the bone. Lame sensation of the wrists and ankles. Strained ankle. Strained back. Pain in nape, back and loins. Backache improves with pressure and lying on back. Lumbago worse morning before rising. Pain from back down hips and thighs Ganglion on wrist. Pain and stiffness in wrists and hands. Pain in bones of feet and ankles. Hamstrings feel shortened. Aching pain in tendo-achilles. Great restlessness. *Ruta* has reputation for improving vision, like *Euphrasia*. It is also excellent for tired, strained eyes. Eyestrain with burning in eyes; maybe followed by a headache. **Symptoms worsen:** Over-exertion. Eye strain. Lying. Sitting. Cold. **Symptoms improve:** Warmth. Gentle motion. Lying on back.

SEPIA

(Ink of the Cuttlefish)

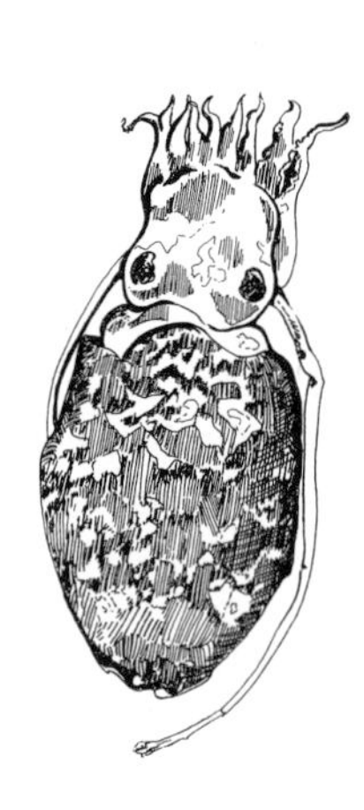

This medicine is well known for its beneficial effects on women's problems. It works particularly well on women who are sallow complexioned, tired, irritable and indifferent to family and loved ones. Mean and spiteful to husband and children. Shouts at or hits children. Resents demands made on them. Feels overworked, unappreciated and taken for granted. Wishes to escape from domestic duties. Loss of femininity in women. Low libido. Exhaustion. Feeling of indifference to life and to family. Life seems colourless - like a sepia photograph. Always busy (must do something useful). Feels emotionally better after vigorous exercise. Anxiety about money. Fears poverty. Stressed and exhausted by the struggle to survive. Loves dancing and aerobic exercise. Fears of poverty, snakes, and rape. Loves storms.

AILMENTS AND SYMPTOMS: Often wears black or brown. Sallow and skinny or overweight, blonde. Brown patches on face (hormonal). White spots on nails. May cry while telling symptoms. Weakness and tiredness worse from 3 p.m. to 5 p.m. Faintness or tiredness while standing. Aversion to sex. Premenstrual tension, with bearing-down feeling in uterus. Pains during sex. Periodic thrush. Dryness of vagina during menopause. Prolapse of uterus, bladder or rectum. Breasts shrivelled. Left-sided headaches, improves with vigorous exercise, worse during menses. Nausea worse in the morning, better from eating. Morning sickness. Stomach feels like a bottomless pit. Eats and eats without satiety. Constipation with feeling of pressure. Back pains worse during menses and from stooping. Vitiligo (main remedy). Herpes around genitals or lips. Dry, scaley and patchy eruptions. Acne during and before menses. Desire for pickles, spices, coffee and chocolate. **Symptoms worsen:** Before and during menses. From foggy conditions, cold air. Pregnancy. Abortion. Sitting, standing, stooping. Before thunderstorms. Ascending. Lifting or straining. Scratching. **Symptoms improve:** With violent exertion. Warm, dry weather. Warmth: of bed. Pressure. Hot applications. Crossing or drawing limbs up. After sleep. Cold drinks; cold bath; open air.

SILICA
(Sand/Quartz)

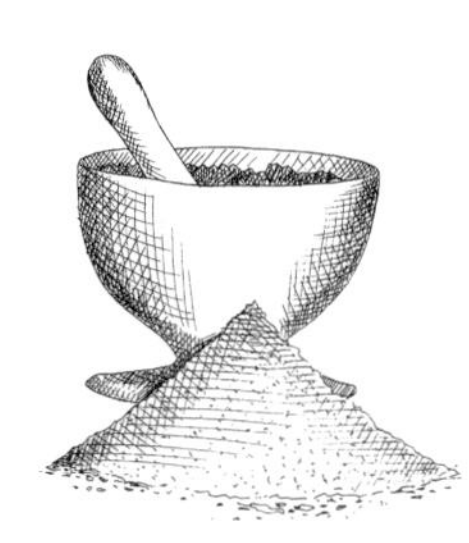

Yielding natures (like sand). Fine hair and transparent skin. Sensitive, gentle and sympathetic people. Artistic and refined. Good at fine, detailed work, such as watercolour painting or architecture. Perfectionist in work. May like dancing and long-distance running. Lack grit at times, at other times persevering. *Silica* strengthens confidence and willpower. Suffer from loss of self-confidence. Fear of social occasions, and of loud or forceful people. Like to please others and to serve others; aware of their needs (*Cocculus*). Healers. Accommodate others too much. Avoid confrontations. Very obstinate if pushed. Anticipation nerves before performance, exams or ordeals. Fear that they will not cope, will fail. Children whiney, clinging, timid. Lack of confidence in delicate children. Very obstinate.

AILMENTS AND SYMPTOMS: Weakness of bones and muscles. Poor spinal development. Sweat on head, palms, and feet. Fine hair and skin. Pale, translucent skin. Large-headed children with small bodies. Nails peel and split. Glandular enlargements. Chronic tonsillitis, or otitis with recurrent discharge from the ears. Boils, abscesses and styes that don't come to a head and discharge their contents. Keloid scars (*Causticum; Graphites*). Cysts. Scoliosis (*Calc Phos; Sulphur*; *Calc Carb*). Constipation. Fibro-adenomas of the breasts. Bunions (*Phosphorus*). Hair falling out with baldness. Milk intolerance. Desires salads and raw foods. Children may eat sand. **Symptoms worsen:** From cold air, draft and damp. From undressing and bathing. Jarring of spine. Moon changes. Night. Mental exertion. Pressure.

Change of weather. **Symptoms improve:** With warm wraps around head. Summer. Wet humid weather. Profuse urination.

STAPHYSAGRIA

(Stavesacre)

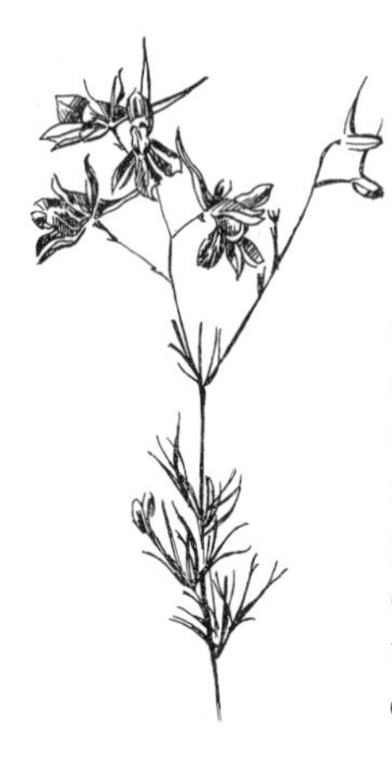

Adults or children who are too nice and accommodating for their own good. Avoid confrontations and don't express anger or assert themselves. Don't stand up for themselves so become victims of circumstance. Often a history of being dominated and abused. Suppress anger and displace it onto safe objects: throw things or abuse weaker individuals, e.g. children. Resentful. Dwell on hurts. Fantasize about what they would like to say, yet lack courage. Cry when confronted or when telling symptoms. Feel unfairly treated. Sensitive to injustice. Easily hurt. Stoical and reserved (*Carcinosin; Nat Mur*). Don't like talking about their problems. Often high sexual desire. Emotional insecurity, jealousy and distrust. Children feel jealous of siblings and unfairly treated. Bouts of violent temper tantrums. Fear of heights, snakes, closed places, poverty, violence, rape.

AILMENTS AND SYMPTOMS: Styes, cysts, tumours. Cystitis, psoriasis and arthritis from suppressed anger. Repeated cystitis, worse after sex or after internalising negative feelings. Arthritis often starts in the fingers. Back pains. Psoriasis after injury. Prostatitis, ovaritis, ovarian cysts, endometriosis. Frontal headaches worse after vexation. Abdominal pain after anger. Addictions - to alcohol, drugs, tobacco, food. Desire sweet, milk and bread. **Symptoms worsen:** From emotions: indignation, vexation, quarrels. Sexual excess. Touch. Cuts or wounds. Surgery. Stretching parts. After urinating; when not urinating. Night. **Symptoms improve:** With warmth. Rest. Breakfast. After sex.

SULPHUR

(Brimstone)

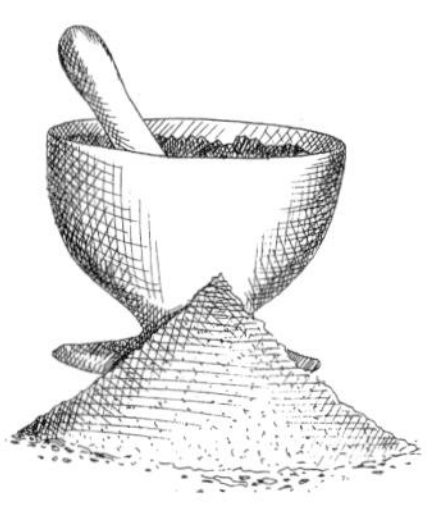

Think of *Sulphur* issuing forth from a volcano. Hot-blooded and hot-headed people. Often creative and artistic or scientific. Inventive: make things and put their hand to many tasks, from building to computer programming. Children invent and make things from an early age. Messy children. Impatient and irritable if held up by traffic or in queues. Hurried, yet often late. Leave things to the last minute. Work under pressure. Go through lazy and untidy spells. Intellectual people with a 'know it all' attitude. Self-centred and opinionated. Critical of others and bossy. Often feel superior to others. Have a little knowledge about a lot of things. Scientists, computer boffs. Anxiety attacks with hurried, irritable, wound-up feeling. May worry about family excessively. Stay up late at night. Work into the early hours. Insomnia. Fears of heights, germs, poverty, failure.

AILMENTS AND SYMPTOMS: Reddish complexion. Red lips or eyelids. Sweat easily. Strong smelling sweat. May be untidy looking. Like wearing old clothes, or dress up with bright colours, particularly red. Burning pains are common. Dry, hot and red skin eruptions. Acne. Burning and itching of eruptions, worse from a hot bath. Burning pains in stomach after eating. Heartburn worse from spices. Offensive stools and gas. Burning in rectum after passing stool. Itching, burning piles. Hot, burning feet; must stick them out. Insomnia: wakes at 5 a.m. and then catnaps. Headaches (worse on weekends). Backache worse standing. Hepatitis. Colitis. Gastritis. Thirsty for water. Likes sweet food or drinks. Likes fried and junk foods. Dislikes vegetables. **Symptoms worsen:** From suppressing eruptions. Becoming heated. Summer. Milk. Noon or mid-morning. Menopause. Standing. Sweets and fats. Looking down. **Symptoms improve:** With open air. Motion. Drawing up affected limbs. Sweating. Lying on right side. Walking.

SYMPHYTUM

(Comfrey or 'Knitbone')

Symphytum is a remedy for injury.

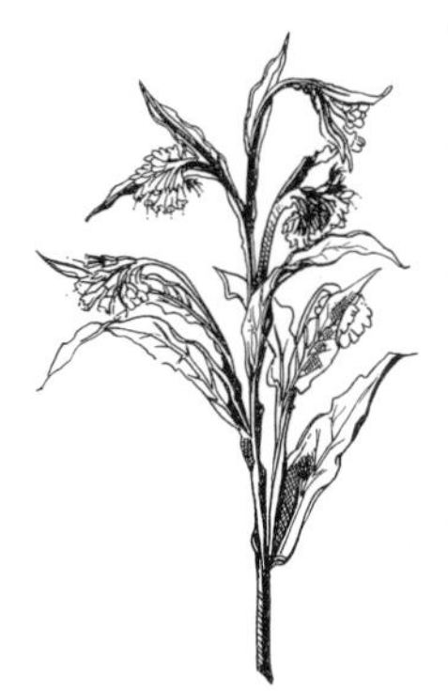

AILMENTS AND SYMPTOMS: It has mainly been used for fractures, both acutely and in cases with non-union of fractures. It is also a useful remedy in injuries to periosteum and bone, with persisting pains long after the injury. It may be alternated with *Ruta*. If alternated with *Calc Phos* it hastens reunion of fractures. It is the specific remedy for trauma to the eyeball with pain remaining. *Arnica* is more useful in injuries to the orbit (surrounding the eye).

THUJA

(White Cypress)

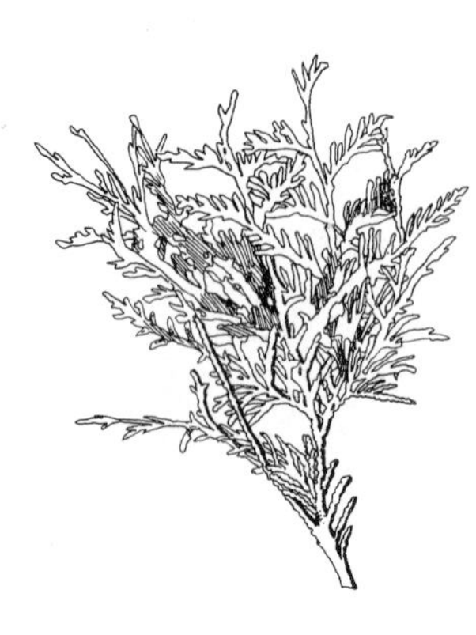

Thuja characters tend to project a pleasant and well mannered front. They are too concerned about what others think of them to let go and behave spontaneously. The 'Christmas tree' front. Too concerned about what others think, secretive and devious. Charming veneer. Like to look good and make a good impression. Dress well, well mannered and polite, except to their family, like *Lycopodium*. (Angel at work, devil at home). Children who are well mannered at school and excitable, quarrelsome or mean at home. Obsessive about appearance (anorexia). Fastidious and controlled. Find it difficult to be spontaneous. Guilt and shame. May dislike themselves, attempting to suppress their natural instincts. Sometimes clandestine double life. Religious fanaticism. Obsessive about diet. Strict and moralistic attitude toward others, and with their children. Poor concentration, drift off during conversation. Feel spaced out, as if in a dream. Hurried for no reason. Sensitive to music. Often musicians or singers.

AILMENTS AND SYMPTOMS: *Thuja* is well known as a remedy for warts. It helps hard and horny little seed warts particularly. *Thuja* counteracts the bad effects of vaccination. It is also important in the treatment of sinusitis, asthma, acne and vaginal discharges. Post nasal drip - hawking. Greasy skin. Red moles. Hard cysts under the skin. Ovarian cysts and fibroids. Left-sided ovaritis. Hair on unwanted parts in women (*Sepia*). Prostatitis (*Staphysagri; Pulsatilla; Conium*). Pain in either iliac area. Sycotic arthritis which is worse from damp. Chronic sinusitis. Asthma worse from damp. Abdominal bloating, with rumbling and gurgling. Desires oranges, bananas, avocado and spices. **Symptoms worsen:** At 3 a.m. and 3 p.m. Sleepiness at 3 p.m. Damp weather. Worse from onions and tea. **Symptoms improve:** Warmth. Air. Discharges. Sneezing. Motion.